Medical Laboratory Statistics

Institute of Medical Laboratory Sciences Monographs

Under the General Editorship of

F. J. BAKER, OBE, FIMLS, FIST, FRMS
*Formerly Principal Medical Laboratory Scientific Officer,
Brompton Hospital, London*

Titles currently available:

Medical Laboratory Statistics by Paul W. Strike
Laboratory Control of Antibacterial Chemotherapy
  by Michael Bryant
Mycobacteria by Maureen V. Chadwick

Some forthcoming titles:

Laboratory Techniques in Immunology by E. T. Davies
Laboratory Investigation of Urine by Ian Leighton
Lymphoid Tissue by G. J. Reynolds
Computer Systems in Medical Laboratory Sciences
  by Paul Ayliffe and Martin Walter
Microbiology in Blood Transfusion by John A. J. Barbara

Medical Laboratory Statistics

Paul W. Strike FIMLS, Dip. Biom., FSS

Biochemist,
R.A.F. Institute of Pathology
and Tropical Medicine

WRIGHT·PSG
Bristol   London   Boston
1981

Published by:
John Wright & Sons Ltd., 42–44 Triangle West,
Bristol BS8 1EX, England.

John Wright PSG Inc., 545 Great Road,
Littleton, Massachusetts 01460, U.S.A.

British Library Cataloguing in Publication Data

Strike, Paul W.
  Medical Laboratory statistics
  1. Mathematical statistics
  2. Medical statistics
  I. Title
  519.5'02461   QA276

ISBN   0 7236 0582 3

Printed in Great Britain by
John Wright & Sons Ltd., at The Stonebridge Press, Bristol BS4 5NU

Foreword

With the rapid advancement of medical laboratory sciences, it is often difficult for the laboratory worker to keep abreast of current knowledge. Major text books cover a wide field of a given major discipline, but obviously they cannot cover every facet of a subject.

The Institute of Medical Laboratory Sciences Monograph Series is written by experts in specific areas, to expand on a subject and to give it the depth and breadth not generally possible in a major work. These books will be useful to those working in the medical laboratory sciences field, for use on the bench, as an examination reference book and for keeping up with current thinking.

I am delighted to have been offered the General Editorship of this series and hope it will be the success it well deserves to be. It is hoped that the Monograph series will be extant for a long period of time and that it will build up to be a useful and welcome addition to your library.

F. J. Baker
London 1981

Preface

The content of this slim volume has been to some extent determined by first-hand experience of the midnight blood barbiturate. What seemed important then and in the small hours of the night is reflected in what follows. The selection is personal, a blend of workshop manual and contemplative essay, with some sixty illustrations for the numerically faint of heart. The level of mathematics demanded never passes beyond simple arithmetic, although there is a good deal of it at times. Much of this can be left to a programmable calculator or computer. It is in the framework of ideas and assumptions within which the trivial arithmetic is performed that the real difficulties lie.

Read this book from cover to cover. Do not dip into it until you have read it at least once. The ideas are developed sequentially, and for the most part pictorially. Difficult areas are continually revisited from different standpoints. The subject of regression in particular is dealt with in a detailed manner, given its central role in the measurement process. Given the constraints upon size and the particular emphasis of the monograph on laboratory measurement, the chi-squared tests have been excluded. A clear and inexpensive introduction can be found in Sprent P. (1977) *Statistics in Action*, Middlesex, Harmondsworth; Penguin.

The book covers most of the requirements of the Institute of Medical Laboratory Sciences Fellowship examinations, and should prove useful to candidates for the Association of Clinical Biochemists Mastership in Clinical Biochemistry, the Royal College of Pathologists Membership examinations and to anyone concerned with the medical laboratory.

It is a pleasure to acknowledge the help of Wing Commander S. A. Cullen of the Royal Air Force pathology branch who had the questionable pleasure of reading everything, much of which never made it to the final draft, thanks to his patient criticism. Professor M. J. R. Healy, of the London School of Hygiene and Tropical Medicine, read an early draft with sharp eye and good humour. My wife Jennifer typed a difficult and ever-changing manuscript, removing a good deal of nonsense on the way.

P.W.S.

Contents

1 Introduction

One thing the scientific discipline of statistics does not lack is a multiplicity of definitions for itself. Barnett (1975) advanced the following provisional definition which seems well suited for this book. Statistics is 'the study of how information should be employed to reflect on, and give guidance for action in, a practical situation involving uncertainty.' It allows us to summarize, manipulate and base inference upon sample data that have an element of uncertainty either as an inherent property or as a consequence of the manner in which they were obtained.

The word 'statistics' has its origins in the collection of information for the State. The military adventures of the 17th century demanded finance and the one main source of this finance, taxation, required a knowledge of taxable assets. 'State information' rapidly infiltrated many of the affairs of government. The 17th century also saw the birth of a new branch of mathematics, probability theory, with its roots in the gaming houses of Europe. In less than a hundred years the approximation of State-istics by probability models was a reality. The development of Statistics owes much to the scientists of the day who recognized its potential importance in their own fields. The astronomer Karl Friedrich Gauss (1777–1855) developed the method of least-squares, a fundamental contribution to the analysis of errors of observation. His essays (recorded in Latin) are a salutary reminder that microprocessors have a long way to go no matter how good a game of chess they may play.

In the past hundred years the science has developed to a considerable level of complexity and subtlety thanks to the contributions of scientists and mathematicians alike. Its reputation has not always matched its substance. In the field of government and economic forecasting in particular it has been, and is seen to be, fallible. Economic situations are complex and for entire nations, the subject of many complex material, social and political interactions. Even after the most exacting statistical analyses, next year remains as much of an unknown quantity as this year was twelve months ago.

1

A second blow to its reputation is paradoxically a reflection on its widespread value. With applications in so many diverse areas—the sciences, economics and industry—it is hardly surprising that a good number of people, armed with any one of the legion recipe books available, attempt their own analyses. The medical journals bear eloquent witness to the quality of many of these enterprises.

Coming to study statistics from a background in the medical laboratory sciences, one is quickly impressed by the contrast between the simplicity of the calculations and the complexity of the reasoning. If you can add two and two you will soon find your way through the arithmetic of a t-test. The logical principles underlying the rejection of one hypothesis in favour of another, on the basis of that t-test, are by no means as easy to grasp; indeed, experts still find the subject an ever ready source of argument and controversy.

Numbers are tricky customers at the best of times. Completely non-existent problems can be conjured out of the most innocent situations simply by adopting the wrong point of view. The following paradox, borrowed from Northrop (1975) is a trivial example of the point. Three men dining together at a restaurant receive a bill for £30. Each man gives the waiter £10 who returns to the cash desk. Here he is told that a mistake has been made over the bill, which should have been £25. He is given £5 to return to the men. Returning to their table, the waiter reasons that £5 is an awkward amount to divide between three men and they of course would be only too pleased to get anything back at all, so, he pockets £2 and gives each of the men £1. Now, each man has paid £9 for his meal. Three times nine is twenty-seven. The waiter has two pounds in pocket. Twenty-seven plus two is twenty-nine. The men originally handed over thirty pounds. Where is the missing pound?

The explanation is obvious given a moment's reflection. Lose this problem in a mass of superfluous facts and figures and the necessary re-orientation may be a lot more difficult to achieve. The point being made is lent a rather chilling reality by the following story, first related by Dr Richard Asher (1954). An investigator observed that of 200 epileptic subjects studied, 24% had infantile convulsions in their first two years of life. Of 200 'normal' subjects only 2% had infantile convulsions in this period. The investigator reasoned that, given the very obvious difference between the 24% in epileptics and the 2% in normals, convulsions in the first two years of life could be taken as strong evidence of epilepsy and the child placed immediately on anti-convulsant therapy.

It sounds plausible but something has been overlooked. Can you detect the fallacy at this point?

No mention has been made of the incidence of epilepsy in the population at large! This is approximately 1:400. In a group of 40 000 people from the general population we would expect to find approximately 100 epileptics, 24 of whom would have had infantile convulsions before they were two years old. However, among the 40 000 people we would also expect to find approximately 800 people, who did not have epilepsy, who also had infantile convulsions before they were two years old, i.e. 2% of 40 000. If we had followed this investigator's advice we would have ended up putting 800 children on long-term anti-convulsant therapy, only 24 of whom actually had epilepsy!

If this example is submerged in another two or three thousand words of text the fallacy may, once again, be far from obvious.

Modern computing devices will effortlessly perform the arithmetic; without a degree of thought they will as effortlessly lead you into trouble. The more complex the problem, the more care you will need to employ in considering both the properties of your observations (e.g. are they *really* a random sample? ... what are they a random sample of? ... are the observations contaminated by measurement errors?) and of your statistics. The computer can calculate correlation matrices for multivariate analyses in seconds, a task that in the past demanded many hours (sometimes months!) of awesomely monotonous calculation. The potential for complete dislocation from any sort of reality in these extremely complicated models is enormous. If you do not have a pretty good idea of where you are, what you are doing and where you want to go before you load the computer, the subsequent journey through a multidimensional vector space may leave you with some substantial illusions, all to ten or more decimal places!

Statistical encounters in the medical laboratory are of more fundamental importance than you might at first admit. The laboratory has much in common with manufacturing industry, processing raw materials to produce a 'product' in response to consumer demand, the product in this case being a 'result'. It is sobering to reflect for a moment upon the body of consumer legislation that would come to bear upon the laboratory if its product were bags of crisps! As it is, the extent to which the laboratory's product, its results, satisfy its main consumer, the clinician, depends upon how well they reflect the clinical reality· Success here depends entirely upon how thoroughly the laboratory has aswered such questions as: 'How do we know we are measuring what we believe we are measuring? . . . How reproducibly do we measure whatever it is we believe we are measuring? . . . How does the inherent variability of our observations affect their diagnostic value?' These and similar questions are often quite profound. A good deal of both common-sense and statistical expertise may be called upon to provide answers that are useful and seen to be useful.

Common-sense is not within the gift of this slim volume and statistical expertise is the substance of an undergraduate discipline.

Between the two lies an awareness of what can be done and what cannot, but often is done.

Most, if not all, laboratory staff have acquired a profound suspicion of any science that ends all of its statements with $p < 0.05$. Years of experience have taught that if there is less than a 1:20 chance that a component will fail, then it will fail in an emergency. The explanation is simple. The $p < 0.05$ was based on an ill-defined sample space. Redefine the problem and you will get the correct answer of $p = 1.0$, i.e. the component will fail in every emergency! This volume will teach you all this and much besides.

REFERENCES
Asher R. (1954) Straight and crooked thinking in medicine. *Br. Med. J.* 2, 460–462.

Barnett V. (1975) *Comparative Statistical Inference*. New York, Wiley.

Northrop E. P. (1975) *Riddles in Mathematics*. Harmondsworth, Middlesex, Penguin.

2 First Steps

2.1 GETTING THE PICTURE

A variable is a property with respect to which individuals in a sample differ in some ascertainable way. Biological variables may be classified as follows:

1. *Nominal*. Also referred to as categorical, attribute or qualitative variables. These cannot be measured or ranked but are expressed qualitatively, e.g. pregnant or non-pregnant. When combined with frequencies they can be treated statistically.

2. *Ordinal*. These have an ordering or ranking significance and nothing more, e.g. the order in which ten eggs hatch; A, B, . . . J. The difference between egg A and egg B has no meaning in terms of magnitude. Sometimes nominal data may be coded in ordinal form. If the nominal variables are responses to a drug, i.e. worse, same, better, much better, they could be coded 1, 2, 3 and 4, each value representing a qualitative improvement on its predecessor.

3. *Measurement*. These have a magnitude significance, i.e. four is twice as great as two. They are divisible into:

   a. Discrete measurement variables: these can assume certain fixed numerical values only with no intermediate values. In practice this implies a count;

   b. Continuous measurement variables: these represent observations on a continuum (length, optical density, etc.) and theoretically an infinite number of values are realizable between any two points. In practice, limitations in the resolving power of the measuring instrument lead to the expression of continuous measurement variables in discrete form, e.g. a blood glucose concentration may be 5·078 913 . . .mmol/l: the assay method is accurate to 0·1mmol/l as a consequence of its imprecision, obliging us to express the blood glucose in discrete form, 5·1mmol/l. The underlying continuum is of considerable importance in subsequent statistical analyses.

Table 1 presents the realizations of a continuous measurement variable, the serum level sof human placental lactogen (HPL) in mg/l for 300 healthy women of child bearing age between 36 and 39 weeks of pregnancy. They were obtained over a twelve month period from five hospitals in different regions of England.

Table 1. Sample of human serum placental lactogen concentrations in 300 women between 36 and 39 weeks of pregnancy.

5·0	6·2	7·1	5·5	6·5	4·6	6·3	8·0	8·5	7·2
7·1	4·0	6·6	7·6	7·9	9·1	10·2	6·3	8·3	5·4
7·8	7·8	6·8	8·5	7·6	5·1	6·6	8·5	7·4	8·7
5·8	9·1	6·2	9·1	9·6	5·8	8·7	10·2	5·7	6·6
7·2	6·9	4·7	5·5	5·7	8·5	5·7	7·8	8·3	6·9
5·4	9·1	7·3	8·0	11·2	7·8	4·3	5·4	7·6	4·8
7·7	8·7	8·7	8·0	6·6	9·6	7·4	6·9	6·6	6·8
8·3	5·3	11·2	9·6	6·3	10·2	5·3	10·2	6·5	6·2
7·3	10·0	9·1	5·8	7·3	6·9	5·8	8·3	4·4	8·5
6·8	9·1	7·1	6·6	5·7	6·3	5·7	8·9	8·5	7·1
9·1	5·8	8·5	12·3	5·7	7·4	7·9	5·8	7·3	11·2
4·5	9·6	10·2	9·8	5·4	6·8	8·0	8·7	6·0	6·3
6·9	10·0	6·0	6·9	7·8	4·9	7·8	8·3	7·3	6·5
4·6	6·6	5·3	11·8	7·3	6·8	9·6	4·6	5·7	8·3
8·5	8·5	9·6	6·5	9·6	7·6	5·0	6·8	5·3	9·6
6·5	7·1	11·5	7·8	6·3	7·1	6·2	6·5	7·8	10·3
5·0	8·5	13·2	11·5	6·0	7·3	8·3	4·0	4·4	8·0
7·8	8·1	9·4	5·5	7·8	7·6	9·4	7·8	7·8	9·4
8·1	6·9	7·8	8·7	5·8	10·5	4·5	5·5	6·3	5·7
7·4	6·6	7·7	13·2	7·4	8·5	8·5	6·3	8·0	7·8
6·5	5·7	6·6	6·2	7·6	6·6	11·4	8·5	7·1	5·5
8·3	10·0	12·7	7·4	12·9	8·7	7·6	4·7	9·6	6·8
7·4	7·8	9·1	6·5	6·3	5·1	9·4	11·2	11·2	6·5
5·4	7·4	12·1	12·3	8·7	8·9	7·8	5·7	11·5	5·8
6·8	6·6	8·7	13·5	7·9	6·8	12·6	10·0	9·6	7·1
6·3	7·6	5·8	4·5	6·6	11·2	11·3	14·0	7·3	10·0
8·9	10·7	5·7	12·1	14·0	6·2	5·3	7·6	6·5	8·1
5·6	7·1	9·8	8·5	12·6	10·5	9·6	8·3	9·1	7·8
9·8	9·8	4·8	10·7	8·1	11·2	9·7	6·8	7·1	9·3
8·0	6·8	10·7	8·1	10·6	6·5	7·1	8·3	6·3	8·9

A casual inspection of the figures reveals very little about the structure of the data. At best we might suggest that most of the values seem to be below ten and they are all rounded to one decimal place. Unravelling the patterns in the data (if any) and summarizing its properties in a few easily interpreted numerical measures may be all that is required. If a more complex analysis is planned these preliminaries will still be necessary in order to ascertain which techniques are appropriate, given the particular properties of the data at hand. A simple histogram may be so telling that subsequent analyses are made unnecessary.

A statistical analysis of the data in *Table 1* presupposes a question in need of an answer. It cannot be emphasized strongly enough that the formulation of this question, whatever it may be, is the most important step in the analysis. It will determine what data is required, how they should be collected and how they should be subsequently treated to give the greatest chance of answering the question unambiguously. Collecting data in the vague hope that an interesting question will suggest itself is rarely productive. Remember the aphorism 'Chance favours the prepared mind'.

For the moment we will assume nothing more than an interest in the HPL data in its own right. Does it have any recognizable structure and can this be used to derive a convenient and informative summary of the data? A statistical shorthand for *Table 1* if you like!

The first step is the preparation of a frequency table for the data. The highest and lowest values in *Table 1* are identified and the range they span divided into a convenient number of equally spaced intervals or classes. Ten to 20 intervals are generally recommended, the exact number chosen depending on the type and quantity of data available. Samples of less than 50 might justify the use of less than 10 classes, whilst samples of 1000 or more may well benefit from the use of more than 20 classes.

The intervals should be constructed so as to exclude the possibility of ambiguous allocations. When the data represent counts this difficulty does not arise.

Number of amoebic forms per mm^3	Frequency
1–4	
5–8	
etc.	

Intermediate values between 4 and 5 cannot occur. When dealing with continuous variables an arbitrary dividing point between two adjacent intervals must necessarily form the upper limit of one class and the lower limit of the other.

HPL	Frequency
4·0–5·0	
5·0–6·0	

To which interval do we allocate HPL values of 5·0mg/l? The problem is simple to resolve but does make for some cumbersome terminology. Any measurement involves an element of approximation. An HPL concentration of 5·0mg/l implies a value in the range of 4·95–5·05. Analytical imprecision obliges us to round off our results to one decimal place, e.g. from 4·95 to 5·0. The continuous variable, HPL concentration, is rendered artificially discrete in that no values between 4·9 and 5·0 are recorded. *Class limits* can be simply defined such that values between or equal to those limits are allocated to that class:

Class limits HPL mg/l	Frequency
4·0–4·9	
5·0–5·9	
6·0–6·9	

Although the class limits are unambiguous with reference to the sample data, problems are raised by the discontinuity of the limits when it comes to drawing a histogram of the data (*Fig. 1*).

We are supposed to be dealing with a continuous variable! Although the class limits are all that is generally shown in published frequency tables and histograms, a second set of limits is operational in the construction of histograms. These are the implied class limits or *class boundaries*, which take into account the underlying approximation in the recorded data by expanding the class limits into the next place of decimals, thereby restoring the underlying measurement continuum.

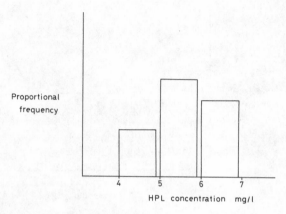

Fig. 1. Histogram defining class limits.

Class limits	Class boundaries	Frequency
4·0–4·9	3·95–4·95	
5·0–5·9	4·95–5·95	
6·0–6·9	5·95–6·95	

Histograms should always be scaled on the class boundaries. If, as is commonly the case, only the class limits are shown, the histogram bars should be drawn a little to the left of the class limits to emphasize the underlying class boundaries (*Fig. 2*).

The frequency table includes two extra columns in *Table 2*. The proportional frequency is obtained by dividing each class frequency by the total number of observations recorded (in the HPL example, 300). This scales the histogram to an overall area of one, considerably simplifying the comparison of histograms based on different numbers of observations. The last column, the cumulative proportional frequency, is obtained by successive addition of the proportional frequencies. The last value will always be 1·00 if the arithmetic is sound. The cumulative proportional frequency has a useful role in assessing the distributional properties of the data, an application referred to in Chapter 4.

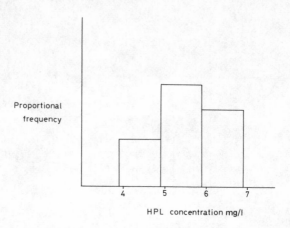

Fig. 2. Histogram defining class boundaries.

If a particular class or classes have very few observations in them they can be pooled. This also serves to 'smooth' out irregularities in the histogram although care should be exercised if valuable information is not to be smoothed into oblivion.

Table 2. Frequency table for HPL values of *Table 1*

Class limits	Class boundaries	Frequency	Proportional frequency	Cumulative proportional frequency
4·0– 4·9	3·95– 4·95	16	0·053	0·053
5·0– 5·9	4·95– 5·95	41	0·137	0·190
6·0– 6·9	5·95– 6·95	61	0·203	0·393
7·0– 7·9	6·95– 7·95	60	0·200	0·593
8·0– 8·9	7·95– 8·95	49	0·163	0·756
9·0– 9·9	8·95– 9·95	30	0·100	0·856
10·0–10·9	9·95–10·95	17	0·057	0·913
11·0–11·9	10·95–11·95	13	0·043	0·956
12·0–12·9	11·95–12·95	8	0·027	0·983
13·0–13·9	12·95–13·95	3	0·010	0·993
14·0–14·9	13·95–14·95	2	0·007	1·000
		$n = 300$	1·000	

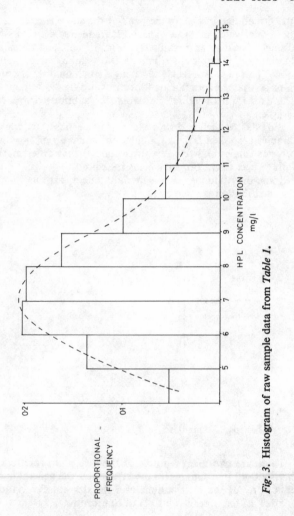

Fig. 3. Histogram of raw sample data from *Table 1.*

A frequency table for the HPL results of *Table 1* is presented in *Table 2* and the corresponding histogram plotted in *Fig. 3*. If the general shape of the histogram is approximated by a curve (the dotted line in *Fig. 3*), the peak of the curve is referred to as the modal value or *mode*. The HPL frequency distribution has a single peak of approximately 7·0mg/l, i.e. it is a unimodal distribution. Sample distributions can exhibit more than one mode. This may be a result of having a small number of observations so that random fluctuations throw up the occasional peak. This is a form of 'noise' and would be suppressed in a larger sample.

Bimodal frequency distributions may be observed when the samples are taken from a 'population' made up of two distinct sub-sets (males and females, for example) that differ markedly with respect to the property being measured.

Some distributions have a modal value at zero as in *Fig. 4*. The distribution is referred to as J-shaped.

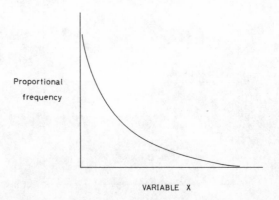

Proportional frequency

VARIABLE X

Fig. 4. J-shaped distribution.

There are two main features of the histogram (or frequency distribution) that summarize the HPL data: the general location or 'centre' of the distribution; and the degree of variation or 'scatter' of the observations about that centre.

2.2. CENTRAL TENDENCY
The arithmetic mean is well known as the sum of the observations divided by the total number of observations. If the HPL variable

is denoted by X, the 300 observations in *Table 1* can be denoted by:

$$X_1, X_2, X_3, \ldots X_n, \text{ where } n = 300.$$

The term X_i is used to denote the HPL variable in general. The arithmetic mean $\overline{X}$ is calculated as:

$$\overline{X} = (X_1 + X_2 + X_3 + \ldots + X_n)/n$$

or more concisely as:

$$\overline{X} = \left(\sum_{i=1}^{n} X_i \right)/n, \text{ where } \sum_{i=1}^{n} \text{means}$$

add up all the X values from 1 to n. This is often abbreviated to:

$$\overline{X} = (\Sigma X_i)/n \text{ or } (\Sigma X)/N. \tag{2.1}$$

For symmetrical distributions the arithmetic mean is the most useful and efficient measure of central tendency. The histogram in *Fig. 3* is however, far from being symmetrical. The right hand 'tail' of the histogram is much longer than that on the left.

The distribution is said to be 'skewed', in this case a right-hand or positive skew. Two other measures of central tendency are applicable to asymmetric distributions: the mode, which we have already described, and the median. The mode is not widely employed in statistical analysis. *The median* is obtained by arranging the observations, e.g. HPL values, in ascending order of magnitude and then locating the value which has an equal number of observations above and below it. For a symmetrical distribution the mean, median and mode are identical (*Fig. 5*).

The mean is considerably more efficient than the median as a measure of central tendency since it utilizes all of the observations in its calculation. The median utilizes only one value (the 'middle' value) and takes no account of the exact magnitude or 'location' of the remainder; it is inefficient in utilizing the 'information' content of the data. For symmetrical or near symmetrical distributions the arithmetic mean is the measure of choice. For highly asymmetric distributions the mean may prove

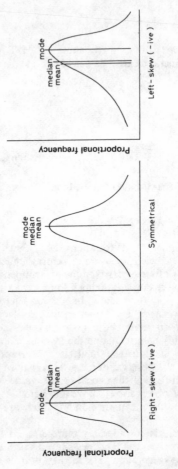

Fig. 5. Effects of asymmetry on measures of location.

misleading, being susceptible to the presence of extreme values in the skewed tail. The insensitivity of the median to anything except the central value now becomes a positive virtue in its role as a descriptive statistic.

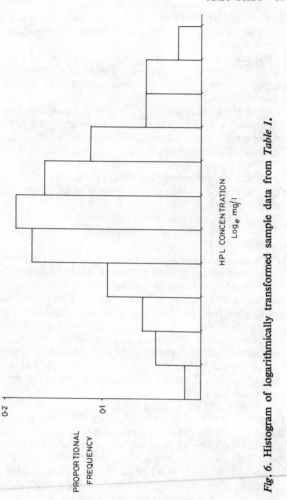

Fig. 6. Histogram of logarithmically transformed sample data from *Table 1.*

The median is not the easiest of quantities to manipulate mathematically, unlike the mean.

The skewed HPL distribution presents us with something of a dilemma. We would prefer to use the arithmetic mean (calculated as 7·78 mg/l) as a measure of central tendency, but the distribution is perhaps ill-suited for its use. An added complication will certainly arise when it comes to describing the spread of the distribution.

The positive skew is suggestive of a log-Normal distribution, i.e. data whose logarithms are Normally distributed. The only property of the 'Normal' distribution that is of interest for the moment is that it is symmetrical.

All of the HPL results in *Table 1* were transformed to natural logarithms. Logarithms to the base$_{10}$—or any other base for that matter—will do just as well. The log-results were then treated like any other set of results in preparing a suitable frequency table and histogram, illustrated in *Fig. 6*.

The distribution of the log-HPL values appears to be a good deal more symmetrical, the arithmetic mean of the log values being 2·01974.

2.3. SCATTER

If you were asked to devise your own measure for the variation of the observations around the mean, it is conceivable that your thinking might proceed as follows:

The range. Why not simply note the maximum and minimum values observed? This is simple to obtain and is expressed in the original scale of the measurements, e.g. mg/l for the HPL variable. Its main disadvantage is similar to that of the median: it utilizes very little of the information available in the data—that of only two observations in fact. This makes the range highly susceptible both to random fluctuations at the extremes of the distribution and to the sample size.

The next line of thought might take the calculation of the arithmetic mean as a starting point. We want a measure of scatter and we want to employ every observation in its calculation. Why not calculate the 'average' scatter around the mean itself? Every HPL result X_i will deviate from the arithmetic mean $\bar{X}$ by a certain amount. If all of the deviations are added up and divided by the total number we will have the mean deviation:

$$\text{Mean deviation} = [\Sigma (X_i - \bar{X})]/n.$$

An immediate problem with this basically good idea is, that for a symmetrical distribution there should be as many positive (+ ive) deviations as there are negative (− ive) ones, so that the term $\Sigma(X_i - \overline{X})$ will tend to zero, leaving us with an overall answer of zero. We could ignore the signs and take the absolute values of the deviations $|X_i - \overline{X}|$.

The term $|X_i - \overline{X}|$ is called the modulus of $X_i - \overline{X}$.

$$\text{Mean absolute deviation} = [\Sigma|X_i - \overline{X}|]/n. \qquad (2.2)$$

This is mathematically clumsy. A cleaner way of getting rid of the negative signs is to square them, which leads to the mean square deviation, or *variance*:

$$\text{Mean square deviation (variance)} = [\Sigma(X_i - \overline{X})^2]/n. \qquad (2.3)$$

This quantity plays a central role in statistical theory. The upper term, $\Sigma(X_i - \overline{X})^2$ is called the sum of squares about the mean. For our purposes the variance is difficult to interpret as a simple measure of scatter. There is much to be said for returning it to the original scale of the measurements, e.g. mg/l by taking its square root:

$$\begin{array}{l}\text{Root mean square deviation}\\ \quad (\textit{standard deviation}) = \sqrt{[\Sigma(X_i - \overline{X})^2]/n}. \qquad (2.4)\end{array}$$

Although the term standard deviation is a good deal easier on the tongue, the rather more elaborate root mean square deviation tells us a good deal more about its origins. Standard deviations calculated on sample data are often denoted by the letter S.

The greater the scatter of the obervations X_i around the mean $\overline{X}$, the greater will be the value of S. The idea is illustrated in *Fig. 7*, which incidentally makes a point of how expensive it can be to reduce the observed variation in a 'manufacturing' process.

Later discussion on the properties of the 'Normal' distribution will reveal that the mean ± 2 standard deviations encompasses approximately 95% of the observations. We will make use of this fact to summarize the log HPL distribution of *Fig. 6*.

The mean of the log HPL values = 2·01974 log mg/l.

The standard deviation = 0·25391 log mg/l.

Approximately 95% of the log HPL values fall in the range $2·01974 \pm (2 \times 0·25391) = 1·51192$—$2·52756$mg/l.

This is all very clever, but we are really interested in the HPL values of *Table 1*, which are in mg/l, not in their logarithms. The

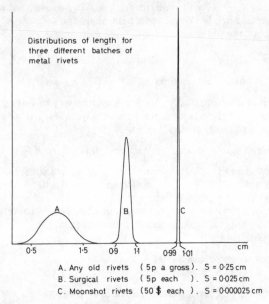

Distributions of length for three different batches of metal rivets

A. Any old rivets   (5p a gross). S = 0·25 cm
B. Surgical rivets (5p each   ). S = 0·025 cm
C. Moonshot rivets (50 $ each). S = 0·000025 cm

Fig. 7. The standard deviation as a measure of scatter.

use of logarithms is simply a device for dealing with the otherwise difficult problems presented by the skewness of the original figures. To return to the original scale of measurement we simply find the appropriate antilog of 1·51192–2·52756, i.e. 4·54–12·52mg/l. Note how this range is asymmetric around the original arithmetic mean of 7·78mg/l.

The antilog of the mean of the log HPL values, 2·01974, gives us 7·54mg/l. This is somewhat lower than the arithmetic mean of 7·78mg/l. The explanation needs to be remembered.

Remember that the addition of logarithms is equivalent to finding the product of the original values:

$$\frac{\Sigma \log X_i}{n} = \frac{\Pi X_i}{n},$$

where $\Sigma \log X_i = \log X_1 + \log X_2 + \log X_3 + \ldots + \log X_n,$

$$\Pi X_i = \quad X_1 \times X_2 \times X_3 \times \ldots \times X_n.$$

The operation $\Pi X_i/n$ gives us the geometric mean, which is always lower than the arithmetic mean (unless all the X_i are identical).

The results of *Table 1* can now be summarized in a convenient statistical shorthand. 95% of the values in *Table 1* fall in the range 4·5–12·5mg/l, these being concentrated asymmetrically around a geometric mean of 7·5mg/l The arithmetic mean is 7·8mg/l.

2.4. FINAL WORDS

Transformations are of considerable value in the statistical analysis of data but they require a good deal of careful thought. For the majority of statistical analyses a number of important properties will be assumed for the data. Transformation of the data to make one assumption true, e.g. to obtain a symmetrical distribution, may invalidate one of the other assumptions in the process, e.g. additive measurement errors may be transformed into multiplicative errors. The more complicated the transformation the more difficult it becomes to assess its consequences on the validity of the analysis.

A second problem arises in transforming the *results* of the analysis back into the original scale of the observations. The appearance of a geometric mean in the log-transformed HPL data bears witness to the potential problems.

The standard deviation of expression 2.4 is more commonly seen with $n–1$ as a divisor. The reason for this is discussed in Chapter 7.2, but a simple explanation for the curious follows.

So far our interest has been confined to the description and summary of a sample of observations in their own right. The standard deviation was employed as little more than an exercise in summary arithmetic. In reality we are not usually interested in the data we have so much as in the data we do not have. We have a set of observations $X_1, X_2, X_3, \ldots, X_n$ but what we want to know is something about the observation X_{n+1}. The sample is only of interest for what it tells us about the world at large, i.e. the 'population' from which it was drawn. *If* a sample standard deviation is used to say something about the variation in the body of data from which the sample was drawn (rather than just the sample itself), a sampling bias is encountered in the mathematics that necessitates the use of a correction factor, taking the form of $n–1$ as a divisor. For samples of sixty or more observations the bias becomes negligible.

A simpler expression for the standard deviation that is algebraically identical to expression 2.4 (with $n-1$ as a divisor) can be used for routine calculations:

$$S = \sqrt{(\Sigma X_i^2 - [\Sigma X_i]^2/n)/(n-1)}. \tag{2.5}$$

Descriptive statistics can convey a great deal about the properties of the data being examined and recent years have seen a considerable resurgence of interest in what might be termed 'data reduction' techniques, i.e. 'getting the facts out of the numbers'. Certainly, anyone who has been confronted by one of *those* tables, crammed with numbers to the exclusion of any empty space (or sense) at all must have wondered what it was the author was trying to convey. A lighthearted look at the presentation of data by Huff (1973) can be recommended; it will save you from many a blunder, and the occasional deceit.

REFERENCES
Huff D. (1973) *How to Lie with Statistics*. Harmondsworth, Middlesex: Penguin.

3 Probability

3.1. INTRODUCTION

Probability is a concept that most of us understand intuitively; we often refer in day-to-day conversation of the 'chance' of a certain event occurring. This view can be formally stated as:

A number between 0 and 1 (or 0 and 100% if you prefer it) that reflects the long term proportion of the number of times a particular event occurs.

The more often we throw a coin, the closer the proportion of tails we get approaches 0.5. Thrown an infinite number of times the proportion will tend to a limit of 0.5, this *limit* being the probability of obtaining tails in any particular throw of the coin (or a more formally, in any particular realization of the coin-throwing experiment).

At the heart of this idea is the concept of a random sequence. In the coin-throwing experiment this sequence would be the recorded heads or tails for a given number of throws of the coin. A random sequence is completely unpredictable, the result obtained for one throw of the coin having absolutely no effect whatsoever on the result of the next throw. The outcome of any one throw of the coin is completely *independent* of any other throw of the coin. Having thrown eight tails in a row, the probability of getting heads on the ninth throw remains 0.5 despite an irrational belief that it must be very nearly inevitable!

Some sequences exhibit random-like behaviour, but in fact the events are linked, often over a period of time. The outcomes are not independent of each other. A simple example is that of Brownian motion, the apparently random agitation of small particles in solution due to the constant bombardment by solvent molecules. The position of a particular particle at any given point in time is to some extent dependent upon its position the moment before. It was of some interest to physicists to calculate the average distance a particle moved from its starting point in a given time. The 'drunken walk' problem was solved by Einstein, who proved that the distance travelled by the particle was proportional to the square root of the time taken. Such 'random-

21

like' sequences are referred to as 'stochastic' processes from the Greek 'stochos' meaning a target. A 'stochastiche' was a person who foretold the future!

The frequency concept of probability is by no means the only one. Many events that are the subject of uncertainty occur in circumstances that are anything but repeatable. The condition of a particular patient at 3 o'clock tomorrow afternoon can hardly be regarded as a random 'sample' from endless repetitions of this event. We are only interested in that particular patient and that particular afternoon. We may believe, on the basis of our experience and knowledge of the case, that the patient is going to become critically ill. The strength or degree of belief that we have in the truth of that opinion could conceivably be quantified. 0 — the patient will not be critically ill; 1 — the patient will be critically ill. If we are 75% sure he will be ill then our subjective probability for this event is 0·75. This represents our *degree of belief* in the truth of the event. The logical basis of subjective probability and for that matter, the frequency concept of probability, remains a subject of often heated debate in mathematical and philosophical circles. The use of subjective probability will be referred to later in this chapter, but for the most part the discussion in this book will presume a frequency model. Methods based upon frequency models have the distinct advantage of having been around for many years so that their shortcomings are well known.

3.2. PROBABILITY RULES

The rules governing the manipulation of probabilities can be considered in the context of some simple experiments.

Experiment: A single coin is thrown four times and the occurrence of heads (H) or tails (T) is noted in the order they occur.

Table 3. Outcome

e_1	H	H	H	H		e_9	H	T	T	H
e_2	H	H	H	T		e_{10}	H	T	H	H
e_3	H	H	T	T		e_{11}	H	H	T	H
e_4	H	T	T	T		e_{12}	T	H	H	T
e_5	T	T	T	T		e_{13}	T	T	H	T
e_6	T	T	T	H		e_{14}	T	H	T	T
e_7	T	T	H	H		e_{15}	H	T	H	T
e_8	T	H	H	H		e_{16}	T	H	T	H

There are sixteen possible results (or outcomes) for this experiment, labelled e_1 to e_{16} in *Table 3*.

This list of all the possible outcomes is called the *sample space* of this particular experiment. The sum of all the possible outcomes in a sample space has a probability of 1·0. This is really stating the obvious in a rather formal way: every time the experiment is performed one of these outcomes *must* occur. We will ignore the possibility of a coin landing on its edge or getting swallowed by a magpie in flight. If you really considered these to be serious possibilities the sample space would clearly have to be modified to accommodate them.

For the sake of clarity *this* coin never gets lost and never lands on its side! If all the outcomes are equally likely then the probability of observing any one of them in the experiment described is 1 divided by the total number of possible outcomes, e.g. the probability of getting four tails in a row is 1/16 or 0·063 or 6·3%.

3.3. CONDITIONAL PROBABILITY

Consider a survey in which a number of subjects are taken at random from a defined population and a note made of whether they are DEAF (A) or DUMB (B). The results of such an imaginary survey are presented in *Fig. 8*.

The proportion of dumb subjects amongst those who also happen to be deaf is described by the frequency ratio f(A and B)/f(A), the limit of which is the probability of being dumb *given* that we already know the subject to be deaf:

Probability of being DUMB
given being DEAF $= p$ (B|A)
$= p$ (A and B)/p (A). (3.1)

The term p (B|A) is called the *conditional* probability of B (being dumb). Suppose that a new subject is taken, at random, from this same population and we are told nothing at all about the state of the individual's hearing. What is the probability that the subject is dumb? From *Fig. 8* the best estimate we can give is 1%:

$$p \text{ (DUMB)} = 0·01.$$

Suppose now that we are given some 'extra information' about this subject, i.e. that he/she is known to be deaf. We can

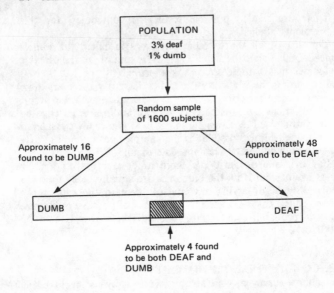

$$\text{Proportion of DUMB subjects in complete sample} = \frac{\text{Number DUMB}}{\text{Total number of sample}} = \frac{f(B)}{N} = \frac{16}{1600} = 1\%$$

$$\text{Proportion of DUMB in sub-sample of DEAF subjects only} = \frac{\text{Number both DEAF and DUMB}}{\text{Number DEAF}} = \frac{f(A \text{ and } B)}{f(A)} = \frac{4}{48} = 8 \cdot 33\%$$

Fig. 8. Hypothetical population study involving two *non-independent* variables.

now regard the subject as a random sample from the *sub-population* of deaf people, and within this sub-population the incidence of dumbness is considerably greater at 8·33%:

$$p \text{ (DUMB|DEAF)} = 0 \cdot 0833.$$

The probability of being dumb appears to be *dependent* on whether or not we know the state of the subject's hearing. The rather abstract but important concept of statistical *independence* can be made accessible if we consider a different population in which the incidence of dumbness is exactly the same amongst deaf subjects as it is for any other member of that population, i.e. 1%. The 'extra information' that a randomly selected subject is deaf would now be of no value at all in re-assessing the probability of the subject being dumb. It remains at 1%,

$$\text{i.e. } p\,(\text{DUMB}|\text{DEAF}) = p\,(\text{DUMB}),$$
$$\text{or} \qquad p\,(\text{B}|\text{A}) = p\,(\text{B}). \qquad (3.2)$$

In this last example the probability of being dumb is quite *independent* of whether or not the subject is deaf.

When the conditional probability of an event $p\,(\text{B}|\text{A})$ is equal to its unconditional probability $p\,(\text{B})$, the two events A and B are said to be statistically independent.

Note: It can be reasonably argued that *all* probabilities are to some extent conditional. The probability of obtaining heads on a single throw of a coin is 0·5. Although we write this as $p\,(\text{HEADS}) = 0·5$ we imply $p\,(\text{HEADS}|\text{An unbiased coin, an unbiased throw, no magpies}) = 0·5$. All subjective probability statements are conditional upon what we know or believe about the event being considered.

3.4. THE MULTIPLICATION RULES

What is the probability that in the coin throwing experiment of *Table 3* we will obtain four heads on two consecutive occasions? We will call the first set of four heads A and the second set B:

Probability of 4 HEADS
and 4 HEADS
$$\begin{aligned} &= p\,(\text{A and B}) \\ &= p\,(\text{A}).p\,(\text{B}) \\ &= 0·063 \times 0·063 \\ &= 0·004. \end{aligned} \qquad (3.3)$$

The *simple multiplication rule* of expression 3.3 assumes that the two events considered are independent of each other, as indeed they are. If the events are not independent of each other then the *general multiplication rule*, obtained from a rearrangement of expression 3.1, must be employed:

$$p\,(\text{A and B}) = p\,(\text{A}).p\,(\text{B}|\text{A}). \qquad (3.4)$$

Consider the population survey of *Fig. 8*. We know that being dumb is not independent of being deaf, so that an answer to the question 'What is the probability of a *randomly selected subject* being both deaf and dumb?' demands the use of the general multiplication rule:

$$p \text{ (DEAF and DUMB)} = 0.03 \times 0.0833 = 0.0025.$$

Independence is an important property that should not be lightly assumed. It is a critical requirement for the application of a large number of statistical methods.

Consider this problem. Suppose that we have a defined population in which the incidence of deafness (A) is 3% and the incidence of tuberculosis (B) is 1.5%. What is the probability that a randomly selected individual from this population is both deaf *and* a victim of tuberculosis? We may be tempted to regard these events as independent of each other and use the simple multiplication rule:

$$p \text{ (A and B)} = 0.03 \times 0.015 = 0.0005.$$

A little thought about the matter might lead to a reassessment of this choice. Tuberculosis is commonly treated with, amongst other things, streptomycin. This antibiotic is directly toxic to the 8th cranial nerve and permanent deafness is a serious side effect of streptomycin therapy. It is conceivable that amongst past and present tuberculosis victims there is a higher incidence of deafness than there is in the population at large. To answer the original question we need the conditional probability of deafness given tuberculosis and the general multiplication rule of expression 3.4.

Failure to obtain a truly random sample can lead to failures in the independence assumption. Imagine that you wanted to observe the effects of a drug on a sample of ten 'normal' rats. Reaching into a cage to pull out the first ten you can catch is a sure recipe for problems! The healthy, strong (clever!) rats will elude you whilst the sickly, weak (stupid!) rats will be the first to get caught. The effects of the drug on a weak, unhealthy rat may be quite different to its effects on a healthy rat. There is only one way to obtain a real 'sample' and that is by using an accepted random sampling scheme. These vary in complexity depending on the nature of the problem. Simply numbering the rats from one to a hundred (or however many there are) and selecting ten from a set of random number tables is a good start (Appendix 1, *Table A*). The random numbers are obtained by reading up, down, across or diagonally (forwards or backwards) from the table, starting anywhere you like, the only precaution being to avoid repeating a sequence for any given experiment.

Random errors in the results of clinical assays are often assumed to be independent of each other.

In *Fig. 9a* are shown the random errors associated with a set of serum glucose assays. Given the random error of any one assay result we can say nothing more about the random error of the adjacent sample results other than that they are equally likely to be positive or negative.

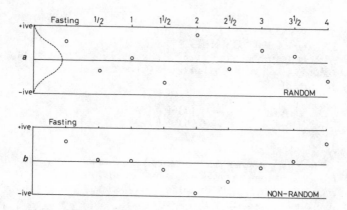

Fig. 9a. Random fluctuations in serial measurements of blood glucose.
b. Non-random fluctuations in serial measurements of blood glucose.

In *Fig. 9b* the random errors exhibit a distinct (cyclic) pattern, possibly due to non-random fluctuations in the analytical conditions. This may be due to reagent deterioration, photocell fatigue or baseline drift on an automated continuous flow analyzer. Given that the random error of one sample result is positive, the probability that the random errors in the adjacent samples are also positive is a great deal higher than 50%. This particular form of dependence (as opposed to independence) is called *serial correlation*. It is a type of stochastic process and can seriously complicate a statistical analysis of the results *as they stand*. If the samples had been assayed in a random order prior to analysis, the subsequent re-ordering of the results (from fasting——→4h) would destroy the effect of the serial correlation.

The within-batch random error of most glucose assay methods is probably small enough to render the example of *Fig. 9a* and *b* of illustrative value only. This cannot be said of hormone assay methods in which random errors *may* be in excess of 20%. Randomization of the test samples prior to assay is absolutely essential if completely spurious 'response' patterns are to be avoided in the results of hormone stimulation and suppression tests.

3.5. THE ADDITION RULES

What is the probability that in the coin throwing experiment of *Table 4* we will get *either* four heads (A) *or* four tails (B) in one experiment?

$$p \text{ (A or B)} \quad = p \text{ (A)} + p \text{ (B)}$$
$$= 0.063 + 0.063$$
$$= 0.126. \quad (3.5)$$

The *simple addition rule* of expression 3.5 requires only that the two outcomes considered cannot occur together. This is clearly impossible in the coin-throwing experiment, but consider the population survey of *Fig. 8*.

We want to know the probability of a randomly selected subject being *either* deaf *or* dumb. We have already observed that $\frac{1}{4}\%$ (0.0025) of the subjects are deaf *and* dumb (from expression 3.4) so that any calculation of the probability of observing one *or* the other must take account of this:

$$p \text{ (A or B)} \quad = p \text{ (A)} + p \text{ (B)} - p \text{ (A and B)}$$
$$= 0.03 + 0.01 - 0.0025$$
$$= 0.0375. \quad (3.6)$$

Expression 3.6 is the *general addition rule*.

3.6. BAYES' THEOREM

Suppose that there was a test for diagnosing a specific type of cancer that gave a positive result in 98% of patients actually having that cancer, and in 4% of patients who did *not* have the cancer.

If 1:200 of the patients in a particular hospital actually had the cancer of interest, what is the probability that a patient selected at random, having a positive test, actually has the cancer?

The sample space for this problem is CANCER | NOT CANCER, for which we have the probabilities $\frac{1}{2}$% and $99\frac{1}{2}$% respectively. The second stage of the problem is the test for which we have the conditional probabilities:

$$p \text{ (+IVE TEST|CANCER)} = 0\cdot98$$
$$p \text{ (+IVE TEST|NOT CANCER)} = 0\cdot04.$$

This information can be summarized diagramatically, *see Fig. 10.*

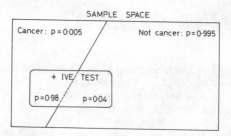

Fig. 10. Sample space for conditional probabilities (cancer *example 3.6*)

We want to know the proability of a patient, drawn at random from this sample space, having the specific cancer, given that his test is found to be positive, i.e. p (CANCER|+IVE TEST).

From expression 3.1 the conditional probability is given by:

$$p \text{ (CANCER| +IVE TEST)}$$
$$= \frac{p \text{ (CANCER and +IVE TEST)}}{p \text{ (+IVE TEST)}} . \quad (3.7)$$

The upper term in expression 3.7 is obtained using the general multiplication rule of expression 3.4 so that it can be re-written as:

$$p \text{ (CANCER} | +\text{IVE TEST)} = \frac{p \text{ (CANCER)} \cdot p \text{ (}+\text{IVE TEST} | \text{CANCER)} \cdot}{p \text{ (}+\text{IVE TEST)}} \quad (3.8)$$

The lower term, p (+IVE TEST) is the *sum* of the probabilities for each partition of the sample space, in the present case these being CANCER and NOT CANCER. More complicated problems can have many more partitions.

$$
\begin{aligned}
p \text{ (}+\text{IVE TEST)} &= [p \text{ (}+\text{IVE TEST} | \text{CANCER)} \cdot p \text{ (CANCER)}] \\
&\quad + [p \text{ (}+\text{IVE TEST} | \text{NOT CANCER)} \cdot p \text{ (NOT CANCER)}] \\
&= (0{\cdot}98 \times 0{\cdot}005) + (0{\cdot}04 \times 0{\cdot}995).
\end{aligned}
$$

Overall we have:

$$p \text{ (CANCER} | +\text{IVE TEST)} = \frac{(0{\cdot}005 \times 0{\cdot}98)}{(0{\cdot}98 \times 0{\cdot}005) + (0{\cdot}04 \times 0{\cdot}995)} = 0{\cdot}11.$$

A randomly selected patient having a positive test has only an 11% probability of actually having the cancer of interest.

You might like to reconsider the epilepsy problem of Chapter 1 in these terms. What is the probability of a randomly selected infant (from the population as a whole) actually having epilepsy, given that it has had infantile convulsions in its first two years of life? (Ans. = 0·003.)

Expression 3.8 is known as Bayes' Theorem and was originally described by the Reverend Thomas Bayes in 1763 in a philosophical essay on probability. As applied above, it is uncontroversial and readily adaptable to much more complicated sample spaces.

More recently, it has been employed in the manipulation of subjective probabilities and here the controversy has been very marked. Reconsider expression 3.8 in the following form:

POSTERIOR PROBABILITY OF CANCER	=	PRIOR PROBABILITY OF CANCER	×	PROBABILITY OF EVIDENCE FOR CANCER

In the example used we knew that the prior probability of cancer for a randomly selected patient was $\frac{1}{2}$%. As a result of performing the test, extra evidence was made available in the form of a positive result. Bayes' theorem allowed us to combine our prior probability with the 'experimental' evidence to revise our estimate of the probability of cancer for that patient. The revised estimate (11%) is called the posterior probability.

The difficulties arise over the prior probability. In the example this was a sound frequency based estimate obtained from previous sample surveys. There are many situations in which a frequency based prior probability is not available, *a* because no one has gone to the trouble of establishing it or *b* because the event being considered does not permit a frequency interpretation.

The success or failure of a new commercial venture (subject to consumer whims and stock market jitters!) is the subject of some uncertainty, but it is hardly a repeatable event. A disease may have certain characteristic features but every patient is different! The businessman and the clinician may, on the basis of their experience and knowledge, believe that a particular situation is more likely than any other. Their subjective assessment of the probability of a particular outcome can be employed as a prior probability. Using Bayes' theorem, this subjective probability can be modified in the light of experimental evidence to provide a refined or posterior probability.

When the experienced judgement degenerates to an inspired (or not so inspired) guess, these *Bayesian* methods become controversial indeed.

The *Frequentist* might argue that if you start off knowing nothing there is no reason to believe you'll be any better off turning your ignorance into numbers. The *Bayesian* would point out that there is nothing so subjective as defining a sample space. Even for such an artificial experiment as throwing a coin four times we quite subjectively chose to regard the possibility of a coin landing on its edge as impossible.

It is reassuring to note that in practice the two approaches generally lead to the same conclusions. The methods of this book are all based on a frequency concept of probability.

4 Probability Distributions

'The map is not the territory'. A. Korzybski

4.1. GETTING THE PICTURE

If we look again at the coin throwing experiment of Chapter 3, we recall that a single experiment consisted of throwing a single coin four times and recording the occurrence of heads or tails for each throw. The list of all the possible outcomes (the sample space) was illustrated in *Table 3*. It would be convenient if this table could be summarized in something like a histogram, and to do this requires the definition of the *random variable* x_i.

In Chapter 2 a variable was defined as a property with respect to which individuals in a sample differ in some ascertainable way. A random variable has an associated frequency (probability) function which determines how often different values occur in the sample space being observed.

For the coin-throwing experiment we define the number of heads observed in any given experiment as the random variable x_i. This could take the values 0, 1, 2, 3 or 4 heads. *Fig. 11* tabulates the frequency of occurrence of the random variable from *Table 3*.

RANDOM
VARIABLE X_i

0	TTTT				
1	HTTT	TTTH	TTHT	THTT	
2	HHTT	TTHH	HTTH	THHT	HTHT	THTH
3	HHHT	THHH	HHTH	HTHH	
4	HHHH				

Fig. 11. Theoretical frequency distribution for the possible outcomes of throwing an unbiased coin four times (H = heads; T = tails).

Each of these outcomes has a probability of 0·063; so we could represent the frequency table in terms of the corresponding probabilities (*Fig. 12*).

RANDOM VARIABLE X_1		Overall Probability
0	$p = 0.063$	$= 0.063$
1	$p = 0.063 + 0.063 + 0.063 + 0.063$	$= 0.252$
2	$p = 0.063 + 0.063 + 0.063 + 0.063 + 0.063 + 0.063$	$= 0.378$
3	$p = 0.063 + 0.063 + 0.063 + 0.063$	$= 0.252$
4	$p = 0.063$	$= 0.063$
		$\overline{1.00}$

Fig. 12. Probabilities associated with the coin-throwing experiment of *Fig. 11*.

The probabilities add up to 1·00 (not exactly, since exact $p = 0.0625$). Turn this table of probabilities through 90° and replace the numbers with bars whose height is proportional to the probabilities; we then have a simple probability distribution (*Fig. 13*).

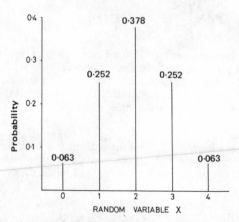

Fig. 13. Probability distribution associated with the coin-throwing experiment of *Fig. 11*.

Sample data histograms such as that of fig. 3 *are essentially approximations to the underlying probability distributions*, the approximation improving as the sample size increases, becoming identical at infinity. If the coin throwing experiment were performed one hundred times and a histogram plotted for x_i (the number of heads in each of the 100 experiments), it would look something like *Fig. 13*. The histogram for one thousand experiments would be very close to *Fig. 13* whilst that for a million such experiments would be very nearly identical.

For the probability distribution of *Fig. 13* the random variable x_i could take only one of five possible values and is referred to as a *discrete* random variable. The particular distribution considered is a Binomial distribution, and it is amongst the commonest of the counting distributions.

4.2. THE BINOMIAL DISTRIBUTION

This is a characteristic distribution for experiments made up of a fixed number of *independent* 'trials', each of which can have only one or two possible outcomes, e.g. for the coin experiment we had four 'trials' (throws of the coin) each with an outcome of *either* heads *or* tails. The probability that the random variable X_i will take a particular value in any given experiment is given by:

$$p(X) = \begin{bmatrix} n \\ x \end{bmatrix} \cdot p^x \cdot (1-p)^{n-x}, \qquad (4.1)$$

where $n =$ the number of trials and $p =$ the probability of obtaining a particular outcome (e.g. heads) in one trial. Expression 4.1 looks a lot more fearsome than it in fact is. The term $\begin{bmatrix} n \\ x \end{bmatrix}$ is called the Binomial coefficient and is best explained by its use in the following example.

Example 4.1

A drug is effective in 75% of the patients to whom it is administered. What is the probability that three out of the next five randomly selected patients will respond to the drug?

$n = 5$
$p = 0.75$
$x =$ number of patients who respond to the drug, i.e. 0, 1, 2, 3, 4 or 5.

$$p(0) = \begin{bmatrix} 5 \\ 0 \end{bmatrix} \cdot (0 \cdot 75)^0 \cdot (0 \cdot 25)^5 = \qquad\qquad (0 \cdot 25)^5 = 0 \cdot 001$$

$$p(1) = \begin{bmatrix} 5 \\ 1 \end{bmatrix} \cdot (0 \cdot 75)^1 \cdot (0 \cdot 25)^4 = \qquad\qquad 5 \cdot (0 \cdot 75) \cdot (0 \cdot 25)^4 = 0 \cdot 015$$

$$p(2) = \begin{bmatrix} 5 \\ 2 \end{bmatrix} \cdot (0 \cdot 75)^2 \cdot (0 \cdot 25)^3 = \qquad \frac{5 \times 4}{2 \times 1} \cdot (0 \cdot 75)^2 \cdot (0 \cdot 25)^3 = 0 \cdot 088$$

$$p(3) = \begin{bmatrix} 5 \\ 3 \end{bmatrix} \cdot (0 \cdot 75)^3 \cdot (0 \cdot 25)^2 = \quad \frac{5 \times 4 \times 3}{3 \times 2 \times 1} \cdot (0 \cdot 75)^3 \cdot (0 \cdot 25)^2 = 0 \cdot 264$$

$$p(4) = \begin{bmatrix} 5 \\ 4 \end{bmatrix} \cdot (0 \cdot 75)^4 \cdot (0 \cdot 25)^1 = \frac{5 \times 4 \times 3 \times 2}{4 \times 3 \times 2 \times 1} \cdot (0 \cdot 75)^4 \cdot (0 \cdot 25) = 0 \cdot 395$$

$$p(5) = \begin{bmatrix} 5 \\ 5 \end{bmatrix} \cdot (0 \cdot 75)^5 \cdot (0 \cdot 25)^0 = \qquad\qquad 1 \cdot (0 \cdot 75)^5 \qquad = 0 \cdot 237$$

$$\Sigma p = 1 \cdot 000$$

Note that $\begin{bmatrix} 5 \\ 0 \end{bmatrix} = 0$ and $\begin{bmatrix} 5 \\ 5 \end{bmatrix} = 1$.

Answer

In answer to the original question, the probability that three out of the next five patients treated will respond to the drug is 0·264. Consider the following manipulations:

p (exactly 3 responding)   = 0·264
p (more than 3 responding)   = $1 - p$ (3 or less)
                          = $1 - (0 \cdot 264 + 0 \cdot 088 + 0 \cdot 015 + 0 \cdot 001)$
                          = 0·6320
p (up to and inc. 3 responding)
                          = $(0 \cdot 264 + 0 \cdot 088 + 0 \cdot 015 + 0 \cdot 001$
                          = 0·368.

Note how the overall probability associated with the distribution = 1·0.

You might like to try your hand at calculating the probabilities of none, one, two, three or four heads in the coin throwing experiment, using expression 4.1. The answers should be close to those in *Fig. 12*, allowing for a little rounding error.

In practice the Binomial distribution becomes increasingly symmetrical as the probability approaches 0·5, and/or as the number of trials involved increase. Consider the distribution for the drug responses with a probability of 75% and five patients (trials), and then again with fifty patients (*Figs. 14a* and *b*).

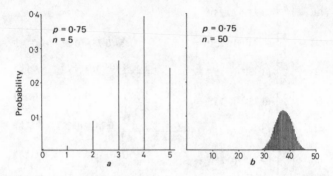

Fig. 14. Increasing symmetry of the binomial distribution as the number of trials increases (and/or *p* approaches 0·5).

The mean of the Binomial distribution is given by $n \cdot p$

The standard deviation is given by $\sqrt{n \cdot p \cdot (1 - p)}$

For the example in *Fig. 14b*, the mean is $50 \times 0.75 = 37.5$ and the standard deviation is $\sqrt{50 \times 0.75 \, (0.25)} = 3.06$.

4.3. THE NORMAL OR GAUSSIAN DISTRIBUTION

When the number of independent trials becomes infinite, the distribution finally becomes quite symmetrical for all values of *p*. A little thought about this suggests that the random variable for an infinite number of trials must be a continuum, i.e. we have made the transition from a discrete random variable (a count) to a continuous random variable (a measurement). The best known of the continuous probability distributions (and there are many of them) is a family of curves defined by the Normal probability density function. Although the mathematics associated with Normal (or Gaussian) distribution are complicated, the curves are completely summarized by only two simple values.

The *location* of the distribution is described by the arithmetic mean; whilst the *spread* of the distribution around the mean is described by the standard deviation (*S*). The greater the numerical value of *S*, the greater the spread of the distribution (*Fig. 7*).

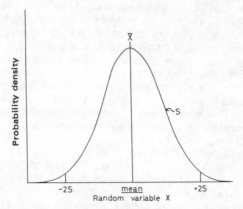

Fig. 15. Characteristics of a Normal or Gaussian distribution.

The standard deviation is located on the inflexion point of the Normal distribution curve (the point at which it alters from a convex to a concave shape, marked S in figure 15). The mean ± 2 standard deviations encompasses 95% of the area under the Normal distribution curve. Since the total area under the curve represents a probability of $1\cdot0$, 95% of the area represents a probability of 95%, i.e. the probability of observing a value for x_i outside the range (mean $\pm 2S$) must therefore be 5% or $0\cdot05$.

The word 'Normal' was applied to the distribution in the context of random measurement error. The measurements considered normally exhibit a Gaussian error distribution and the word normal passed into common usage as the name of the distribution itself. There is certainly nothing normal about the Normal distribution apart from its name. It is no more 'conventional, ideal, healthy etc', than the Binomial distribution. In order to avoid any confusion with the common English usage of the word normal, the Normal distribution (in the sense of being Gaussian) will always be referred to with a capital N.

The importance of the Normal distribution is considerable. Although it is not a property of anything in the real, observed world (consider its theoretical extension to infinity at both extremes if you doubt this!) it can be used as an *approximation* of many random variables. The fact that infinitely tall and infinitely small people do not exist does not prevent us using a

Normal distribution as an extremely useful approximation or model for the distribution of height in defined populations. All science is approximation; technology is finding the right level of approximation for the task in hand. Additionally, the 'statistics' calculated on sample data, e.g. sample means and standard deviations, themselves have probability distributions (discussed in Chapter 7) and these are almost invariably Normally distributed even if the original sample on which they were calculated was not. This is a result of the powerful Central Limit theorem which confers upon the Normal distribution a central role in classical statistical theory.

The value of the Binomial distribution was realized in answering questions of the form 'What is the probability of, say, three patients out of the next five treated responding to a particular drug?' When this was increased to 'thirty out of the next fifty?' the total probability of $1 \cdot 0$ had to spread itself over a much larger number of possible results with the probability of any one particular result becoming smaller and smaller. A more practical question in these circumstances might take the form: 'What is the probability of *up to* thirty patients responding to the drug? We could calculate this as the sum of the individual probabilities for each of 0, 1, 2 . . ., 30 patients but the calculations (using expression 4.1) would be incredibly tedious and, for 25 patients and less, would involve some extremely small numbers, e.g. the probability of one response out of fifty, given a 75% success rate, would be $1 \cdot 18 \times 10^{-27}$.

A far simpler approach is to approximate the by now almost symmetrical distribution (*Fig. 14b*) by a Normal distribution. It is not difficult to imagine a smooth, continuous frequency curve superimposed upon the closely packed frequency bars. The immediate advantage is that the technique for calculating probabilities for the Normal distribution is highly developed and extremely simple.

4.4. STANDARD NORMAL VARIABLES

A continuous random variable x_i can theoretically take any one of an infinite number of possible values, each with an infinitesimal probability. Interest is generally confined to calculating the probability of observing values of x_i in certain intervals, e.g. less than 30, between 32 and 37, or, greater than 41.

The probability of any given interval is directly related to the area above that interval. For example, the probability of observing x_i between 52 and 60 units is represented by the shaded area of the distribution in *Fig. 16*.

The area can be calculated by integration (area-finding) of the Normal probability density function. If this function were fixed, a table of the probability integral could be prepared and subsequent integrations performed simply by reference to this table. The problem is that this function is not fixed; it has two variables, the mean and standard deviation, giving rise to an infinite number of possible Normal curves. We are confronted with the problem of integrating an awkward function every time we want to calculate a probability.

The solution to this problem is very straightforward. We prepare tables of the Normal probability integral for a *Standard Normal Variable* for which we define a mean of zero and a variance of one (and hence a standard deviation of one, since $\sqrt{1} = 1$). This standard variable is commonly represented by the symbol N (0, 1).

Given an observed random variable x_i from a Normal distribution with, for example, a mean of 50 and a standard deviation of 6, we calculate the corresponding Standard Normal variable Z_i from the *transformation* of expression 4.2.

$$Z_i = \frac{x_i - \text{mean}}{\text{Standard deviation}} = \frac{x_i - 50}{6} \ . \qquad (4.2)$$

Subtracting the mean shifts the location of the distribution of x_i to zero. This has no effect upon the shape of the distribution, only where it is *located* on the variable scale. Dividing by the standard deviation places the x_i variable on a scale of unit variance, i.e. if x_i was one standard deviation away from the mean, the corresponding value of Z_i would be one. The transformation of expression 4.2 allows us to take observations from any Normal distribution and manipulate them into corresponding Standard Normal variables Z_i for which tables are widely available for probability calculations. Some examples are given below.

Example *4.2*
Find the probability of observing values of x in the range 52–60, the shaded area in *Fig. 16*, given a mean of 50 and a standard deviation of 6.

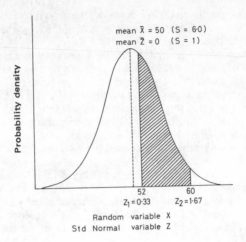

Fig. 16. Example 4.2.

$$\text{If } X_1 = 52, \text{ then } Z_1 = (52 - 50)/6 = 0.33;$$
$$X_2 = 60, \text{ then } Z_2 = (60 - 50)/6 = 1.67.$$

Our problem now takes the modified form: 'Find the probability of observing values of Z_i in the range 0·33–1·67 (*Fig. 16*) given a mean of zero and a standard deviation of 1.

We now refer to Appendix 1, *Table B* for a table of the Standard Normal Integral. Since the Normal distribution is perfectly symmetrical about the mean it is only necessary to tabulate values for one half of the distribution. *Table B* tabulates values from zero (the mean) to four standard deviations to the right of the mean (*Fig. 17*).

The column on the left of *Table B* is headed 'Standard deviation units', i.e. Z_i. Taking Z_1 first we locate the value 0·3 in this column and read across to 0·33. The value tabulated is 0·1293. For Z_2 we find a tabulated value of 0·4525.

The area of the curve between Z_1 and Z_2 (shaded area in *Fig. 16*) is 0·4525 − 0·1293 = 0·3232.

Answer

In answer to the original problem, there is a 32·32% probability of observing a value x_i in the range 52–60 units.

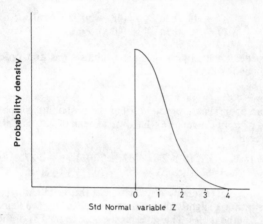

Fig. 17. The area of the standard Normal distribution integrated in Appendix 1, *Table B*.

Example *4.3*

Find the probability of observing values of x_i in the range 40–48 given a mean of 50 and a standard deviation of 6. The problem is the exact mirror image of the first one (*Fig. 18*).

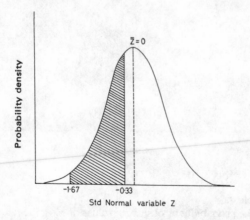

Fig. 18. Example 4.3.

$$\text{If } X_1 = 48, \text{ then } Z_1 = (48 - 50)/6 = -0\cdot33;$$
$$X_2 = 40, \text{ then } Z_2 = (40 - 50)/6 = -1\cdot67.$$

It is dealt with by ignoring the minus signs and proceeding exactly as for the first problem.

Example *4.4*

A more complicated problem. Find the probability of observing values of x_i in the range 67–85 given a mean of 70 and a standard deviation of 11.

$$\text{If } X_1 = 67, \text{ then } Z_1 = (67 - 70)/11 = -0\cdot27;$$
$$X_2 = 85, \text{ then } Z_2 = (85 - 70)/11 = \quad 1\cdot36.$$

The interval covers the central area of the distribution (*Fig. 19*) necessitating a slightly different approach to the problem. Look up $0\cdot27$ in the tables. This gives us the area to the left of the mean (effectively!), i.e. $0\cdot1064$. Now look up $1\cdot36$ to obtain the area to the right of the mean, i.e. $0\cdot4131$. The total area is given by $0\cdot1064 + 0\cdot4131 = 0\cdot5194$. There is a $51\cdot94\%$ probability of observing a value X_i in the range 67–85 units.

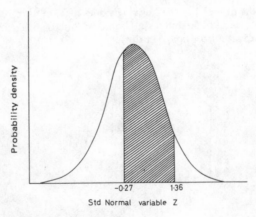

Fig. 19. Example 4.4.

Example *4.5*

Find the probability of observing values of x_i in the range 40–80 units given a mean of 60 and a standard deviation of 10.

$Z_1 = -2 \cdot 0$ and $Z_2 = +2 \cdot 0$. The interval of interest is symmetrical about the mean so we need only look up the integral for $2 \cdot 0$ and double it, i.e. $0 \cdot 4772 \times 2 = 0 \cdot 9544$. This result confirms an earlier statement that the mean $\pm$ two standard deviations encompasses approximately 95% of the area under the Normal curve. *Exactly* 95% of the area is encompassed by the mean $\pm 1 \cdot 96$ standard deviations.

Example *4.6*
As a final example we might pose a question of the form: 'What is the probability of observing values of x_i *up to* 56, given a mean of 60 and a standard deviation of 10 (*Fig. 20*)?'

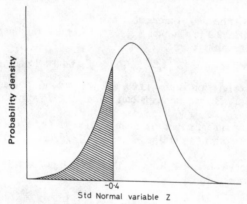

Fig. 20. Example 4.6.

Answer
The question is answered by taking advantage of the symmetry of the distribution and of the fact that the area of one half of the distribution is exactly $0 \cdot 5$. By calculating the area between the mean and the limit of 56 and subtracting it from $0 \cdot 5$ we obtain the answer to the original question.

If $X_i = 56$ then $Z_i = -0 \cdot 4$. The area between the mean and $-0 \cdot 4$ is, from *Table B*, $0 \cdot 1554$. The area left from $0 \cdot 5 - 0 \cdot 1554$, i.e. $0 \cdot 3446$, is that up to $-0 \cdot 4$ (or 56). There is therefore a $34 \cdot 46\%$ probability of observing a value of x_i up to 56 units.

4.5. TESTING NORMALITY
The use of the Normal distribution as an approximation for

summarizing the properties of sample data has already been referred to. A number of different approaches are available for testing whether or not the sample data are compatible with a Normally distributed parent population. To be of any real use most of them require very large samples of data; certainly anything less than 300 samples is going to require some very careful interpretation. You could do a great deal worse than simply plot a reasonable histogram of the data and look at it. If the frequency distribution appears symmetrically bell-shaped around a central mean, a Normal approximation may prove entirely adequate for your purposes. The more important the purpose, the more trouble you should take to model the sample data realistically.

4.5.1. The method of moments
Expression 2.3 in Chapter 2 gave the formula for the variance of a distribution:

$$\text{variance} = [\Sigma (x_i - \bar{x})^2]/n = [\text{Standard deviation}]^2$$

This expression is also known as the 'second moment about the mean'. Higher moments can be calculated from:

3rd moment about the mean $= \mu_3 = [\Sigma (x_i - \bar{x})^3]/n$;
4th moment about the mean $= \mu_4 = [\Sigma (x_i - \bar{x})^4]/n$.

A more convenient form of these equations is available for calculation purposes:

$$\mu_3 = \left[\frac{1}{n} \cdot \Sigma x_i^3\right] - \left[\frac{3}{n} (\bar{x} \cdot \Sigma x_i^2)\right] + 2\bar{x}^3; \tag{4.3}$$

$$\mu_4 = \left[\frac{1}{n} \cdot \Sigma x_i^4\right] - \left[\frac{4}{n} (\bar{x} \cdot \Sigma x_i^3)\right] + \left[\frac{6}{n} (\bar{x}^2 \cdot \Sigma x_i^2)\right] - 3\bar{x}^4. \tag{4.4}$$

These terms are used to calculate the following coefficients:

Coefficient of Skewness $\beta_1 = \mu_3/[\text{Standard deviation}]^3$; \hspace{1em} (4.5)

This coefficient takes the value zero for a Normal distribution—positive values indicate sample data that are skewed to the right, whilst negative values indicate a skew to the left; and

Coefficient of Kurtosis $\beta_2 = \mu_4/[\text{Standard deviation}]^4$. \hspace{1em} (4.6)

For a normal distribution, β_2 takes the value 3. If β_2 is greater than 3, the sample distribution has rather more values in the tail regions than would be expected for a Normal distribution. If β_2 is less than 3, the distribution is more concentrated in the centre than would be expected for a Normal distribution.

For the HPL data of *Table 1*, the coefficients were calculated from equations 4.3 and 4.4 as follows:

$$\Sigma x = 2333\cdot1, \qquad \bar{x} = 7\cdot777,$$
$$\Sigma x^2 = 19\,360\cdot29, \qquad S = 2\cdot013,$$
$$\Sigma x^3 = 171\,143\cdot133, \qquad \mu_3 = 5\cdot560\,17,$$
$$\Sigma x^4 = 1606\,509\cdot289, \qquad \mu_4 = 53\cdot386\,66,$$

from which we obtain $\beta_1 = 0\cdot681\,641$ and $\beta_2 = 3\cdot251\,305$.

Since we are calculating these coefficients on sample data, they will exhibit a certain amount of variability due to the sampling procedure alone, the smaller the sample size the greater the sampling variability. This sampling variation will be just as much in evidence with samples drawn from perfectly Normal population distributions so that the estimated coefficients β_1 and β_2 are unlikely to be exactly 0 and 3 under any conditions. The question that confronts the analyst then is 'how far away from 0 and 3 must the coefficients be before I *reject* the hypothesis that the sample was drawn from a Normally distributed population?'

Taking the coefficient β_1 first, we proceed to answer this question as follows:

Calculate the standard deviation of β_1 (S_{β_1})

for samples of more than 150 $= S_{\beta_1} = \sqrt{6/n}$

for samples of less than 150 $= S_{\beta_1} = \sqrt{\dfrac{6n(n-1)}{(n-2)(n+1)(n+3)}}$

for our sample we have $= S_{\beta_1} = \sqrt{6/300} = 0\cdot141\,42.$

Now calculate the standard Normal variable Z_{β_1} as follows:

$Z_{\beta_1} = (\beta_1 - \text{Expected value of } \beta_1)/S_{\beta_1}$

$\quad = (0\cdot681\,641 - 0)/0\cdot141\,42 = 4\cdot82.$

Our 5% critical value for the test statistic Z_{β_1} is $\pm1\cdot96$, and the 1% critical value is $\pm2\cdot58$. From *Table B* it is easy enough to deduce that the mean of a Standard Normal variable (zero) $\pm1\cdot96$ encompasses 95% of the area under the Standard Normal distribution curve, whilst the mean $\pm 2\cdot58$ encompasses 99% of the area.

The critical values tell us that if samples are randomly selected from a completely symmetrical population, the test statistic Z_{β_1} will be less than $\pm 1\cdot96$ for 95% of such samples, and less than $\pm 2\cdot58$ for 99% of such samples.

Since our test value of $4\cdot82$ is well in excess of the 1% critical value, the probability that our HPL sample was drawn from a symmetrically distributed population (with respect to HPL values), must be rated as quite low (considerably less than 1% in fact). We denote this fact by writing $p < 0\cdot01$ in brackets after the estimated coefficient β_1.

We appear to have good evidence for rejecting the hypothesis that maternal serum HPL is a Normally distributed variable in the population at large (since the Normal distribution is by definition symmetrical). This is a reasonable conclusion if, and only if, we are prepared to accept that our sample data were typical of the population at large. This is a profoundly important aspect of the analysis and receives further consideration in Chapters 5 and 7.

Looking at the coefficient of kurtosis, β_2, we proceed in a similar manner, as follows:

Calculate the standard deviation of β_2 (S_{β_2}).

For samples of less than 1000 this is obtained as:

$$S_{\beta_2} = \sqrt{\frac{24n(n-1)^2}{(n-3)(n-2)(n+3)(n+5)}}.$$

For our sample we have:

$$S_{\beta_2} = \sqrt{\frac{24 \times 300(300-1)^2}{(300-3)(300-2)(300+3)(300+5)}}$$
$$= 0\cdot2805.$$

Now calculate the Standard Normal variable Z_{β_2} as follows:

$$Z_{\beta_2} = (\beta_2 - \text{expected value of } \beta_2)/S_{\beta_2}$$
$$= (3\cdot251\ 305 - 3)/0\cdot2805 = 0\cdot894.$$

The critical values for the test statistic Z_{β_2} are the same as for Z_{β_1}. Since our test value of $0\cdot894$ is well below the 5% critical value of $1\cdot96$, we have no good evidence for rejecting the hypothesis of zero kurtosis in the population distribution, i.e. there is a greater than 5% probability of observing a sample value for β_2 of 3·25 in a sample of 300 HPL values from a Normal population distribution. We would denote this fact by writing $p > 0·05$ in brackets after the estimated coefficient β_2.

Transforming the individual HPL values in *Table 1* to logarithms has the effect of pulling in the right-hand tail values, making the distribution more symmetrical (*Fig. 6*). If we recalculate the coefficients β_1 and β_2 on the transformed data, we obtain:

$$\beta_1 = 0·035\ 989,$$

$$\beta_2 = 2·690\ 132,$$

from which we calculate the test statistics:

$$Z_{\beta 1} = (0·035\ 989)/0·141\ 42 \quad = \ 0·254,$$

$$Z_{\beta 2} = (2·690\ 132 - 3)/0·2805 \ = \ -1·105.$$

Reference to the critical values confirms that both test values are below the 5% critical value, i.e. the observed coefficients do not provide sufficiently convincing evidence for rejecting the hypothesis of Normality for log-HPL concentrations in the population at large. It would appear that the use of a logarithmic transformation *in this case* has been effective in Normalizing the distribution.

Alternative approaches

There are a number of alternative approaches to testing the Normality assumption, these being directed at *general* departures from Normality as opposed to the rather more *specific* tests for skewness and kurtosis.

Probability paper can be employed to plot the cumulative proportional frequencies from *Table 2*, to obtain a *Normal Plot*. Normally distributed data produce a straight-line plot; anything other than a straight-line is indicative of non-Normality. The problem here is one of interpretation, not unrelated to the question: 'How far away from 0 and 3 must the coefficients of skewness and kurtosis be ...?' Sample data from a Normally distributed population will rarely produce a perfectly straight line on probability paper. How much curvature you are prepared to tolerate before you reject the hypothesis of Normality is very much a matter of experience (and sample size).

There is a class of tests known as 'goodness-of-fit' tests. The χ^2-goodness-of-fit test (chi-squared) takes the data of *Table 2* as a starting point. It is a very general test and its 'power' is to some extent dependent upon the number of frequency classes chosen by the analyst. A large number of observations is essential and every frequency class requires an absolute minimum of 5 observations.

The Kolmogorov–Smirnov goodness-of-fit test (K–S test) has no such restriction on sample size and is an attractive technique when sample sizes are unavoidably small.

4.5.2. The modified K–S test

In its original form, the K–S test requires the *population* mean and standard deviation to be known, an impractical requirement for our purposes. The test has been modified by Lilliefors (1967) to deal with the situation in which we have only the *sample* estimates of the mean and standard deviation.

Table 4. Serum assay values: $n = 20$

10·4	4·5	8·2	13·0
3·0	11·0	6·8	8·4
8·9	6·5	5·0	7·0
6·2	7·8	11·6	5·5
7·2	9·3	9·6	9·9

Twenty assay values for a particular serum constituent are given in *Table 4*. We would like to know whether this sample is compatible with a Normal population distribution for that analyte. We make two assumptions which must be valid if the analysis is to be meaningful:

1. That the subjects examined were randomly drawn from the population of interest; and

2. That none of the test results have been discarded for anything other than sound technical reasons.

These assumptions underpin every statistical analysis.

The test protocol follows:

a. Rank the test values of *Table 4* in ascending numerical value.

b. Calculate the mean $\bar{x}$ and standard deviation S (expression 2.5).

c. Transform each of the sample values to their corresponding Standard Normal variables Z_i by subtracting $\bar{x}$ and dividing by S.

d. For each Z_i calculate the cumulative Normal integral f_i as follows:

If Z_i has a negative value, locate the corresponding Normal integral in *Table B* and *subtract* it from 0·5.
e.g. If $Z_i = -1·60$, locate 1·6 in the left-hand column of *Table B* and read across to the column headed 0 (i.e. 0·445). Then
$$f_i = 0·5 - 0·445 = 0·055.$$

If Z_i has a positive value, locate the corresponding Normal integral in *Table B* and *add* it to 0·5.
e.g. If $Z_i = +1·60$, the Normal integral is 0·445 as before, but now
$$f_i = 0·5 + 0·445 = 0·945.$$

e. For each rank calculate the expected value F_i as follows:

F_i = rank number/sample size n.
e.g. if the sample size is 20, F_1 = (1/20) = 0·05,
F_2 = (2/20) = 0·10,
and so on to F_{20} = (20/20) = 1·00.

f. Calculate the absolute differences (i.e. ignore the sign) between f_i and F_i.

g. Note the largest difference recorded as d-max. This is the required test statistic.

Interpretation
Refer to Appendix 1, *Table C* for critical values of the modified K–S test statistic d-max. Locate the sample size $n = 20$ in the left-hand column and read across to the required critical region, e.g. 0·05. The tabulated critical 5% value is 0·190. Since the test d-max of 0·07 (from *Table 5*) does *not* exceed this critical value, we conclude that the sample provides insufficient evidence for rejecting the hypothesis of Normality.

Be quite clear about the implications of this conclusion. It is in no way a 'proof' that the hypothesis is true. We have quite simply failed to extract convincing evidence from the sample data that it is not true. If the test d-max had exceeded the 5% critical value, we would have rejected the hypothesis of Normality, accepting a 5% risk of being wrong in so doing. Chapter 7 deals with these notions in rather more detail.

Table 5. K–S Goodness-of-fit test d-max $= 0.07$

Rank i	Ranked assay values x_i	Z_i $\dfrac{(x_i - \text{mean})}{\text{(std. dev)}}$	f	F $[(1/n) \times \text{rank}]$	d $(|F - f|)$
1	3·0	−1·96	0·03	0·05	0 02
2	4·5	−1·37	0·09	0·10	0·01
3	5·0	−1·18	0·12	0·15	0·03
4	5·5	−0·98	0·16	0·20	0·04
5	6·2	−0·70	0·24	0·25	0·01
6	6·5	−0·59	0·28	0·30	0·02
7	6·8	−0·47	0·32	0·35	0·03
8	7·0	−0·39	0·35	0·40	0·05
9	7·2	−0·31	0·38	0·45	0·07 ←
10	7·8	−0·08	0·47	0·50	0·03
11	8·2	0·08	0·53	0·55	0·02
12	8·4	0·16	0·56	0·60	0·04
13	8·9	0·36	0·64	0·65	0·01
14	9·3	0·52	0·70	0·70	0·00
15	9·6	0·63	0·74	0·75	0·01
16	9·9	0·75	0·77	0·80	0·03
17	10·4	0·95	0·83	0·85	0·02
18	11·0	1·18	0·88	0·90	0·02
19	11·6	1·42	0·92	0·95	0·03
20	13·0	1·97	0·98	1·00	0·02

$$\text{mean} = 7·99$$
$$\text{std. dev} = 2·541$$
$$n = 20$$

If we are interested in testing the more specific hypothesis of whether the sample data were drawn from a *particular* Normal distribution, simply substitute the (known) mean and standard deviation of this distribution for the sample $\bar{x}$ and S at stage *b*, and then proceed as before. The critical value for the test statistic d–max is obtainable from Appendix 1, *Table D*.

REFERENCES

Lilliefors H. W. (1967) On the Kolmogorov–Smirnov test for Normality with mean and variance unknown. *J. Am. Statist. Ass.* **62**, 399–402.

5 Clinical Reference Values

5.1. A QUEST FOR THE FABULOUS NORM

It is a curious fact of laboratory life that the enormous advances in the efficiency with which results are 'manufactured' have not always been matched by an increased understanding of the product itself. Two questions continue to perplex the observer. Is the result accurate and is it normal (clinically)? This is not to say that strenuous efforts have not been made to answer both of these questions. The subject of accuracy will be taken up in Chapter 10.

For the moment then, 'Is it normal?' It is a profoundly important question and often the only one of interest to the doctor who, after all, asked for the test in the first place. He would like a range of values within which he can be reasonably certain that his test is not indicative of disease and outside of which he has reasonable grounds for taking further clinical action. Given that 'normality' in the clinical sense is not un-equivocally defined and bearing in mind the enormous spectrum of clinical and sub-clinical disease, it will surprise no one to learn that any range of the sort described will lead to the occasional incorrect decision. Some subjects who are perfectly healthy will have test results outside of the healthy range of values (a false positive result: a *type I* or α error) and some subjects who are ill will have test results within the 'healthy' range (a false negative result: a *type II* or β error). For the doctor's 'range' to be of practical value *both* types of error should be as small as possible and here we have a classical dilemma. The two types of error sit at the opposite ends of a rather complicated mathematical see-saw (as one comes down . . .!) with the whole construction shrouded in uncertainty as to what exactly constitutes a normal person. Some might argue that we are all sub-clinically ill!

The problem can be resolved into two distinct questions:

1. What population are we going to employ for the purpose of evaluating the 'normality' of a particular test result?

51

2. Given a sample of test results from the particular population decided upon, how do we determine the doctor's 'normal' range?

The vast majority of normal ranges in common use consist of nothing more than two numbers, with little or no information regarding the two questions above. The 'sample' may have been every member of a hospital's staff who had not fallen for the same trick before and the 'range' established by 'statistical' methods for which the word dubious might have been specifically coined.

Wintrobe (1967) has noted that the normal red blood cell counts of 5 and 4·5 million per mm^3 for men and women respectively were based on counts made on only four subjects, over a hundred years ago! These normal values do seem to have been useful. The question is, how much more useful would they have been given a rigorously defined procedure for establishing normal ranges?

The International Federation of Clinical Chemistry (IFCC) have published provisional recommendations on the theory of *Reference values*, the terms involved being set out in *Table 6*.

The original IFCC report can be recommended for a clear and concise description of the Reference value philosophy. The use of the term reference interval implies that each stage in the reference process of *Table 6* has been fully defined for the particular assay concerned. This is intended to distinguish the *reference interval* from the ill-defined *normal range*.

The definitions do not actually do very much to resolve the problems of questions 1 and 2. They simply oblige us to define quite clearly how we resolve the problem ourselves in any particular case.

The first of the two problems, that of defining the reference population, is central to all statistical inference and will be dwelt upon, in that context, in Chapter 7. Suffice it to say that a sample drawn from the healthy laboratory staff of Liverpool may not prove a very sound basis for assessing the normality of an Argentinian cowboy's blood cholesterol, quite irrespective of whether or not the same assay method was employed in each case. It *may not* provide a very sound basis for assessing the normality of blood cholesterols in Liverpudlians unless every patient works in a laboratory. No amount of mathematics can help you here, only observation and experiment!

The second problem, that of defining the reference limits, has received a great deal of attention in recent years with the Normal

(Gaussian) distribution playing an important and controversial role. It is worth repeating here that the Normal probability distribution originated in the description of random errors in repeated measurements on a fixed quantity such as length. The 'true' length was estimated by the arithmetic mean of the repeated measurements, the random errors being symmetrically scattered around the mean in a Gaussian or Normal distribution.

Table 6. IFCC Provisional recommendations on reference value terminology

Reference individuals
  make up a
Reference population
  from which is drawn a
Reference sample group
  on which are determined

Observed values
on a new individual
may be compared
with

Reference values
  which are observed to have
Reference distribution
  from which are calculated
Reference limits
  that may be used to define
Reference intervals

The terms are defined as follows:

A *Reference individual* is an individual selected using defined criteria.

A *Reference population* consists of all possible reference individuals.

A *Reference sample group* is an adequate number of reference individuals selected to represent the reference population.

A *Reference value* is the value obtained by observation or measurement of a particular type of quantity on a reference individual.

A *Reference distribution* is the distribution of reference values.

A *Reference limit* is derived from the reference distribution and is used for descriptive purposes.

A *Reference interval* is the interval between, and including, two reference limits.

An *Observed value* is a value of a particular type of quantity, obtained by observation or measurement, to be compared with the reference values, reference distributions, reference limits or reference intervals.

There is *no* national mean uric acid value around which we are all scattered with 'error'. The variation observed in such biological variables is a consequence of complex biological, genetic and environmental factors peculiar to *each* individual. If such variables happen to be approximately Normally distributed we can take advantage of the fact by summarizing the observed distribution by its mean ± 2 standard deviations. There are certainly no good grounds for supposing that the distributions of these variables should be Normal and very often they are not. The use of the Normal approximation to describe reference distributions is quite opportunist although there are good reasons for using it where it is appropriate. When the reference distribution is obviously non-Normal or where the tests of Chapter 4 reveal it to be so, suitable transformations may be explored that would permit the use of a Normal approximation on the transformed reference values, e.g. the logarithmic transformation of the HPL results in Chapter 2.

If the reference distribution refuses to submit to transformation then a distribution free (or non-parametric) technique such as *percentiles* can be used to describe the distribution. Percentiles are extremely simple in principle and in practice. Simply rank the reference sample values in ascending order of magnitude and define the percentile limits as those sample values beyond which the required percentage of sample values fall at each extreme. For example, if there were a thousand reference sample values, the 2·5th and the 97·5th percentiles would be the assay values of the 26th and 974th ranked specimens respectively.

Assuming that the reference sample *was* drawn from a perfectly healthy reference population, the exclusion of 5% of the values, by whatever method, in defining the reference limits, is equivalent to accepting a 5% false positive error rate in assessing new test results. It would be nice to think that this was the result of a conscious, reasoned decision but the truth is that it is largely historical accident. The Normal distribution, be it appropriate or not, has been the main tool for defining normal ranges in the past. The mean ± 2 standard deviations has a distinct ring of authority to it and has been very widely employed in setting the limits to normal ranges. Well, the standard deviation is no more 'standard' than the Normal probability distribution is 'normal'. If its technical name (from expression 2.4), the 'root mean square deviation', had been used in place of the 'standard deviation', its role in arbitrarily deciding who is 'healthy' and who is not might have been more critically examined. The use of 2·5th and 97·5th percentiles to throw out the 5% healthy extremes is simply a continuation of the 'standard' tradition.

It was remarked that, where appropriate, the Normal approximation is to be preferred to non-parametric methods. The reasons are related to those put forward in Chapter 2 in comparing measures of spread for sample frequency distributions; the range and the standard deviation. Parametric methods make use of every observation in the sample, i.e. they are efficient in utilizing the 'information' contained in the sample. The simpler non-parametric descriptive measures are inefficient, depending on only a few of the observations in the whole sample group. For percentiles to achieve the same sort of efficiency as the Normal approximation (when appropriately applied!) much larger sample sizes are required. Flynn et al. (1974) in a study of 19 biochemical variables in 1000 healthy blood donors found percentiles to be no more than 50% efficient—to attain the same precision in establishing reference limits as that achieved using Normal approximations on suitably transformed assay values, twice as many values would have been required.

A second reason for selling the Normal approximation is the increasing interest in *multivariate* reference values. These will be described a little later but their importance is considerable and their dependence upon the assumption of Normality is very considerable. If the data are Normally distributed on testing then do not hesitate to use the Normal approximation. If they are not, transform them until they are. The paper by Flynn et al. has some useful tips in this direction. If all else fails, use percentiles, but do make sure your reference sample is a big one (300 is an arbitrary but useful minimum!).

Whatever criteria we employ for establishing the acceptable false positive error rate, the false *negative* error rate remains an unknown quantity. All we can be really sure of is that if we push out the reference intervals to reduce the incidence of false positives, the incidence of false negatives will certainly increase. *Figure 21* illustrates the problem.

If reference distributions could be established for healthy subjects *and* for specific disease populations then the exact probability that an observed assay value came from any particular distribution could be calculated using nothing more complicated than the techniques of the previous chapter. Rather

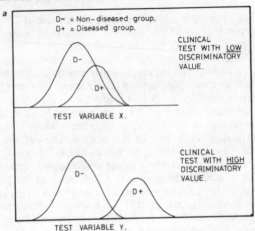

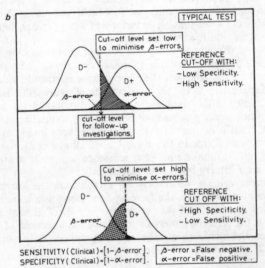

Fig. 21. *The clinical value of test results and their reference intervals.* The clinical *Sensitivity* of a test is a measure of its ability to detect those subjects actually having the disease. The clinical *Specificity* of a test is a measure of its ability to distinguish those subjects not having the disease. The use of these terms is becoming established in the context of screening programmes and clinical decision making. This is unfortunate, given that they have alternative meanings in the fields of analytical chemistry and Bioassay. The false-positive and false-negative error rates are clumsier terms, but they convey the message with a good deal less ambiguity.

more elaborate Bayesian techniques could also be brought into the picture, taking the cancer diagnosis problem of expression 3.8 as a starting point. By reporting the assay result with a range of probabilities for various clinical possibilities, the doctor would be left to make his own decisions as to the 'normality' or otherwise of the patient.* The work involved could be to some extent shouldered by the computer, but, the problems of defining clearly and unambiguously each disease group and establishing pathological reference intervals along the lines of *Table 7* would be quite considerable. That being said, it does seem rather paradoxical to invest considerable capital in producing results and to invest next to nothing (be it time or money) to ensure that they actually mean something. As a basis for clinical action the laboratory result is, given a modicum of reproducibility in the assay method, entirely dependent on the validity of its relation to the reference intervals being employed by the clinician!

5.2. THE 95% PARADOX

For the most part we are obliged to work with simple 95% intervals based on samples from a 'healthy' population (healthy by consensus of opinion!) counting ourselves fortunate if they meet the IFCC requirements. For the assessment of individual assay results they are an imperfect but useful tool. When we come to assess several different assay results on the same patient however, some curious inadequacies are revealed.

Assume that we have a single assay result on a perfectly healthy patient and a 95% reference interval. The probability that the patient's assay value will fall inside the 'healthy' reference interval is 95% or 0·95.

Now assume that we have two quite independent assay values on that same patient, each having its own 95% reference interval. What is the probability that both results will fall within their respective 95% 'healthy' intervals? Recall the *simple multiplication rule* (expression 3.3). The answer to the question is 0·95 × 0·95, i.e. 0·90. In other words there is a 10% probability that *one* of the two assay values will fall outside of its reference interval. The argument is extended in *Table 7*.

---

* A detailed assessment example is given in *Appendix 5A* at the end of this chapter.

Table 7

Number of unrelated assays performed on a healthy individual:

1	2	3	4	5	6	7	8	9	10	11	12	20	40	∞

Probability of obtaining an 'abnormal' result (%):

5	10	14	19	23	26	30	34	37	40	43	46	64	87	100.

One of the more disturbing aspects of *Table 7* is that the demand for independent assays is quite realistic. One might have expected certain groups of assays, such as thyroid function tests, to be anything but independent, but a study by Kagedal et al. (1978) is very revealing. They measured the free thyroxine index, the free triiodothyronine index and thyrotropin levels in 3885 healthy middle-aged women and found that 13·9% had at least one measured value outside of the 95% healthy reference intervals. The expected proportion for three *independent* assays is, from *Table 7*, 14%.

The problem is well known in association with the multiple test profiles delivered by automated analyzers. *Table 7* provides an answer to that most vexing of philosophical questions ... who is normal? The answer is plain—anyone who hasn't been investigated thoroughly enough!

A superficially attractive solution to the problem is to increase the size of the individual reference intervals until all of the probabilities on the lower line of *Table 7* are returned to 5%. For example, if we have a twelve assay profile then readjusting each of the individual reference intervals from the mean ± 2 standard deviations to the mean $\pm 2\cdot 86$ standard deviations reduces the false positive error rate from 46% to 5%. The price paid for this simple exercise is to increase to an unknown extent the false negative error rate for all twelve assays. The paradoxical situation is created in which an assay result which *may* be abnormal in isolation must now be judged normal simply because it was part of a twelve assay profile!

5.3. MULTIVARIATE REFERENCE REGIONS

The problems raised in attempting to interpret groups of individual (univariate) reference intervals have led to experiments

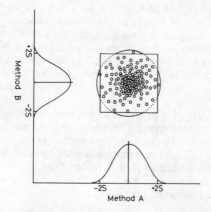

Fig. 23. The multivariate 95% reference *region* (bounded by the circle) for two *independent* assays on one patient.

If the results of the two assays were not independent of each other, e.g. if a high result by assay A tended to be associated with a high result by assay B on a given patient, the bivariate distribution would assume an elliptical shape as in *Fig. 24,* the area encompassed now being considerably smaller than that of the corresponding square:

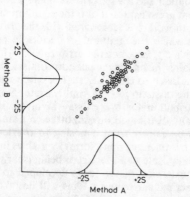

Fig. 24. The effect of non-independent (correlated) assays on the multivariate reference database.

The pairs of results plotted in *Fig. 23* are said to exhibit no correlation. Those of *Fig. 24* exhibit some correlation. Complete correlation of the pairs of results in which the results of assay A were a perfect function of the results of assay B would see the ellipse collapse to a single line with all of the points located on it.

Correlation, the subject of Chapter 8, has really been sneaked in the back door here. Independent variables are uncorrelated variables!

The extension of *Fig. 24* to three variables sees the two-dimensional ellipse become a three-dimensional ellipsoid shape, a 'cloud' of points in the three dimensional graph space if you like. The 95% reference boundary is something like a skin around the 'cloud' of points such that it encloses 95% of the trivariate points. The extension to the four dimensional hyperellipse is best visualized as a mathematical extension of the trivariate ellipsoid.

The calculations involved can be looked at as an extension of the simple univariate case. For a single 95% reference interval we employed the arithmetic mean and the square root of the variance (the standard deviation). For the multivariate calculations we require the mean and variance for each of the assays involved and, additionally, a measure of the correlations between the results of the different assay methods, using a quantity called the covariance. These are employed in a rather elaborate statistical analysis, the end products of which are a set of multi-pliers in an equation and a 95% critical value. The assay results on a new patient are substituted into the equation and the result (it is very easy to work out) compared with the critical value. If it exceeds this value the 'pattern' of results is judged to be 'abnormal' with a 5% false positive error rate. The false negative error rate remains an unknown quantity (unless, as suggested, steps have been taken to establish it). The entire analysis stands or falls on the assumption of multivariate Normality, i.e. a Normal distribution for every assay involved. If the results are not Normally distributed or cannot be so transformed then very little will be gained from choosing to overlook this fact. The statistical treatment of non-Normal variables in this context is extremely complicated and far from being clearly resolved.

A powerful extension of the ideas developed to date is into the field of discriminant analysis. This will be taken up in the chapter on multivariate analysis (Chapter 9) but a few words are in order here.

Imagine that the data points plotted in *Fig. 24* actually describe two populations instead of one healthy one, e.g. healthy subjects and subjects with a fairly well defined disease. A representative sample of subjects from each of the two populations is drawn and two assays, A and B, performed on each member of each sample group. The paired results are plotted in *Fig. 25*.

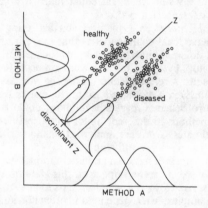

Fig. 25. Extension of the multivariate approach to discrimination between clinical sub-groups.

Looked at from the point of view of assay A or assay B there is a good deal of overlap in the results from healthy and diseased subjects. The discriminant function Z is a linear combination of the results such that the graph is rotated onto a new axis permitting maximum separation of the two groups. In practice the arithmetic is simply adjusted such that a positive value for Z allocates the patient to one group whilst a negative value allocates the patient to the second group.

The example of *Fig. 25* is rather artificial. The discriminant function reveals its considerable power in unravelling half a dozen or more substantially overlapping variables. The analysis can be extended to accommodate allocations to more than two groups and to determining optimum combinations of laboratory tests to obtain the most efficient diagnostic allocations.

5.4. REFERENCE INTERVALS AND THE SINGLE LABORATORY!

Who should establish reference intervals? The answer is, unavoidably, everyone with an assay to perform. There are two primary reasons:

1. The *population* you are dealing with is unique, be it geographically, racially, culturally or in a hundred and one additional ways, any one of which could make a nonsense of an 'imported' reference interval.

2. The *laboratory assay* method you are using will almost inevitably have local characteristics that make it unique. In an ideal world different analytical methods for measuring the same material would, by virtue of their common accuracy, all deliver the same results. A reference interval for one would be a reference for them all. Even a casual glance at the results from national quality control schemes reveals beyond any doubt that the *same* analytical methods in different hands characteristically disagree in their estimates. *Different* analytical methods simply do not measure the same thing, full-stop!

Strenuous efforts at national and international standardization are certainly having some impact on this state of affairs, particularly with regard to the simpler constituents of body fluids. Assays for complex, heterogeneous and often ill-defined materials such as specific proteins, enzymes and many hormones, for which there may be no consensus on standardization or methodology, *must* have locally established reference intervals, updated if needs be to accommodate changes in the assay, e.g. new antibody!

In isolation, the laboratory result is about as useful as a random number. Its clinical value is almost entirely determined by its relation to the reference intervals employed by the doctor. It's a contract from which all the most expensive technology in the world cannot release you.

REFERENCES

Benson E. S. (1972) The concept of the normal range. *Hum. Pathol.* 3, 152–155.

Flynn F. V., Piper K. A. J., Garcia-Webb P. et al. (1974) The frequency distributions of commonly determined blood constituents in healthy blood donors. *Clin. Chim. Acta* 52, 163–171.

Grasbeck R., Siest G., Wilding P. et al. (1978) IFCC Committee on Standards. Provisional Recommendation on the theory of reference values. Part 1. The concept of reference values. *Clin. Chim. Acta* **87**, 459F–465F.

Kagedal B., Sandstrom A., and Tibbling G. (1978) Determination of a trivariate reference region for free thyroxine index, free triiodothyronine index and thyrotropin from results obtained in a health survey of middle-aged women. *Clin. Chem.* **24**, 1744–1750.

Mainland D. (1971) Remarks on clinical "Norms". *Clin. Chem.* **17**, 267–274.

Wintrobe M. M. (1967) *Clinical Haematology*. London, Kimpton.

Appendix 5A:
Clinical Decision Making

5A.1. SCREENING TESTS

Given a serum analyte of which the distributional characteristics
(i.e. reference ranges) are known for the disease states of interest,
estimate the probability that a serum level equal to or greater
than a specified cut-off level X is associated with each disease
state. The distributions of the analyte for three disease states
A, B and C are shown in *Fig. 5A.1*.

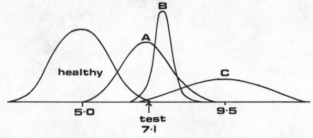

Fig. 5A.1 Decision making under uncertainty

Information Required

a. The *distributional characteristics* of the analyte in the populations of interest. We assume these distributions to be approximated by a Normal (Gaussian) distribution curve, either directly
or by transformation.

Example:

State	Mean	Std. deviation
healthy	5·0	0·9
condition A	6·9	0·8
condition B	7·5	0·4
condition C	9·5	0·85

b. The *prevalence* of the states in the population from which the subject has been drawn. These are the prior probabilities of the states in the absence of additional qualifying information on that subject. If the patient possesses some history, sign or symptom identifying him as being at greater risk than usual, the prevalence data required would be for the 'at-risk' sub-population. For example, in screening for fetal Neural Tube Defects (NTDs), history of a previous NTD-affected pregnancy substantially alters the NTD prevalence rates for the mother concerned.

Example:

State	Prevalence or prior probability
healthy	0·99500
condition A	0·00002
condition B	0·00318
condition C	0·00180

Note how the distributions in *Fig. 5A.1.*, presented with no scale on the *y*-axis, distort the population picture by taking no account of the above prevalences, i.e. the probability density scale is in fact different for each of the distributions shown. Drawn to scale, distributions A, B and C would be vanishingly flat relative to the 'healthy' distribution.

Information Given

Required screening cut-off level for serum analyte = 7 units.

We assume that the assay method used in the screening programme is the same as that used in establishing the reference data *and* that the imprecision of the measurements is essentially unchanged. With this assumption, no account need be taken of analytical imprecision in the following calculations since this error is already incorporated in the reference data themselves.

Calculations

(i) Calculate the Standard Normal deviate for each state:

$$Z_{norm} = (7 - 5·0)/0·9 = 2·2222$$
$$Z_A = (7 - 6·9)/0·8 = 0·1250$$
$$Z_B = (7 - 7·5)/0·4 = -1·2500$$
$$Z_C = (7 - 9·5)/0·85 = -2·9412$$

(ii) Calculate the area under each Normal curve, to the right of the *Z* values, using *Table B*, Appendix (*see* Chapter 4, section 4.4). These areas will be termed 'likelihoods'.

$$\textit{Likelihood}$$

$$L\,(Z_{\text{norm}}) = 0{\cdot}5 - 0{\cdot}486\ 87 = 0{\cdot}013\ 13$$
$$L\,(A) \quad = 0{\cdot}5 - 0{\cdot}049\ 74 = 0{\cdot}450\ 26$$
$$L\,(B) \quad = 0{\cdot}5 + 0{\cdot}394\ 35 = 0{\cdot}894\ 35$$
$$L\,(C) \quad = 0{\cdot}5 + 0{\cdot}498\ 37 = 0{\cdot}998\ 37$$

(iii) Use Baye's theorem (expression 3.6) to revise the prior probabilities in light of a test value equal to or greater than 7 units. The calculations are set out in two stages to simplify the presentation.

a. Multiply the prior probabilities by the likelihoods from step (ii), and obtain the sum:

$$\textit{Prior} \times \textit{Likelihood}$$
$$0{\cdot}995\ 00 \times 0{\cdot}013\ 13 = 0{\cdot}013\ 07$$
$$0{\cdot}000\ 02 \times 0{\cdot}450\ 26 = 0{\cdot}000\ 01$$
$$0{\cdot}003\ 18 \times 0{\cdot}894\ 35 = 0{\cdot}002\ 84$$
$$0{\cdot}001\ 80 \times 0{\cdot}998\ 37 = \underline{0{\cdot}001\ 80}$$
$$\text{Sum} = \overline{0{\cdot}017\ 72}$$

b. Obtain the *screening posterior* probabilities as (Prior × likelihood)/Sum:

p [Unaffected|Test value = 7 units or more]
$$= 0{\cdot}013\ 07/0{\cdot}017\ 72$$
$$= \underline{0{\cdot}7377}\ (73{\cdot}8\%)$$

p [Condition A|Test value = 7 units or more]
$$= 0{\cdot}000\ 01/0{\cdot}017\ 72$$
$$= \underline{0{\cdot}0006}\ (0{\cdot}06\%)$$

p [Condition B|Test value = 7 units or more]
$$= 0{\cdot}002\ 84/0{\cdot}017\ 72$$
$$= \underline{0{\cdot}1603}\ (16{\cdot}0\%)$$

p [Condition C|Test value = 7 units or more]
$$= 0{\cdot}001\ 80/0{\cdot}017\ 72$$
$$= \underline{0{\cdot}1016}\ (10{\cdot}2\%)$$
$$\text{Sum} = 1{\cdot}000$$

The sum of the posterior probabilities should be 1, a check on the arithmetic. The posterior probabilities represent the risk of a test subject having any one of the conditions A, B or C given a test value of 7 or more. They are best described as *screening probabilities*, of value in defining the most effective cut-off levels for a screening programme; the cut-off level of choice would be that providing the optimum trade-off between healthy individuals subjected to expensive/or high risk follow-up investigations, and unhealthy subjects who remain undetected in the screening programme.

Screening probabilities have very little to contribute to the interpretation of individual test results. They are primarily a management tool of use in defining an efficient screening programme.

Having identified an 'at-risk' subject, e.g. with a test value of 7·1 units, the assessment of the posterior probabilities associated with that individual test value requires a slightly different approach.

5A.2. INDIVIDUAL RISK ASSESSMENTS

These are generally of more interest to clinicians faced with a test result on a particular individual. What is the probability that a specific test value, e.g. 7·1 units, is associated with any one of the disease states A, B or C?

The information requirements are similar to those of section 5A.1.

Calculations

(i) Calculate the Standard Normal deviate for each state:

$$
\begin{aligned}
Z_{norm} &= (7{\cdot}1 - 5{\cdot}0)/0{\cdot}9 &=& \quad 2{\cdot}333\,3 \\
Z_A &= (7{\cdot}1 - 6{\cdot}9)/0{\cdot}8 &=& \quad 0{\cdot}250\,0 \\
Z_B &= (7{\cdot}1 - 7{\cdot}5)/0{\cdot}4 &=& -1{\cdot}000\,0 \\
Z_C &= (7{\cdot}1 - 9{\cdot}5)/0{\cdot}85 &=& -2{\cdot}823\,53
\end{aligned}
$$

(ii) Calculate the height of each Normal curve at the Z values. The height, or probability density $f(Z)$, is obtained as:
$$f(Z) = 1/[\sqrt{(2\pi)} \times \exp{(Z^2/2)}].$$
By way of example we will calculate the probability density associated with Z_{norm}.

$$
\begin{aligned}
f(Z_{norm}) &= 1/[\sqrt{(2\pi)} \times \exp{(2{\cdot}3333^2/2)}] \\
&= 1/[2{\cdot}5066 \times \exp{(2{\cdot}7221)}] \\
&= 1/38{\cdot}15 \\
&= 0{\cdot}02622
\end{aligned}
$$

The results are:

$$
\begin{aligned}
&\qquad\qquad \textit{Likelihoods} \\
&f(Z_{norm}) = 0{\cdot}026\,22 \\
&f(Z_A) \quad\;\; = 0{\cdot}386\,67 \\
&f(Z_B) \quad\;\; = 0{\cdot}241\,97 \\
&f(Z_C) \quad\;\; = 0{\cdot}007\,41
\end{aligned}
$$

(iii) Multiply the prior probabilities by the likelihoods and obtain their sum:

$$
\begin{array}{l}
Prior \times Likelihood \\
0{\cdot}995\,00 \times 0{\cdot}026\,22 = 0{\cdot}026\,09 \\
0{\cdot}000\,02 \times 0{\cdot}386\,67 = 0{\cdot}000\,008 \\
0{\cdot}003\,18 \times 0{\cdot}241\,97 = 0{\cdot}000\,77 \\
0{\cdot}001\,80 \times 0{\cdot}007\,41 = \underline{0{\cdot}000\,012} \\
\qquad\qquad\qquad\quad Sum = \overline{0{\cdot}026\,88}
\end{array}
$$

Obtain the individual posterior probabilities as (Prior × Likelihood)/Sum.

p [Unaffected|Test value   = 7·1 units exactly]
$$\qquad\qquad\qquad = 0{\cdot}026\,09/0{\cdot}026\,88$$
$$\qquad\qquad\qquad = \underline{0{\cdot}9706}\ (97{\cdot}06\%)$$
p [Condition A|Test value = 7·1 units exactly]
$$\qquad\qquad\qquad = 0{\cdot}000\,01/0{\cdot}026\,88$$
$$\qquad\qquad\qquad = \underline{0{\cdot}0003}\ (0{\cdot}03\%)$$
p [Condition B|Test value = 7·1 units exactly]
$$\qquad\qquad\qquad = 0{\cdot}000\,77/0{\cdot}026\,88$$
$$\qquad\qquad\qquad = \underline{0{\cdot}0286}\ (2{\cdot}86\%)$$
p [Condition C|Test value = 7·1 units exactly]
$$\qquad\qquad\qquad = 0{\cdot}000\,01/0{\cdot}026\,88$$
$$\qquad\qquad\qquad = \underline{0{\cdot}0005}\ (0{\cdot}05\%)$$
$$\qquad\qquad\qquad Sum = 1$$

These 'individual' probabilities are notably different from the screening probabilities for values of 7 or more, but they are in line with common-sense. Borderline test-values imply borderline risks!

The above procedures can be applied to assessing risks for any number of disease states, given the availability of distributional data (reference ranges) for each state considered, along with the prevalence of those states in the population under study.

5A.3
An important area of application for these methods is the screening of maternal serum and amniotic fluid alpha-fetoprotein (AFP) levels to identify pregnancies 'at-risk' of being associated with fetal neural-tube defects (NTDs). Mothers with serum AFP levels in excess of specified screening cut-off levels are subjected to amniocentesis and the risk of carrying an NTD affected fetus reassessed from the observed amniotic fluid AFP level.

The most efficient cut-off levels for the primary serum screen are established using the screening probability assessments of section 5A.1. Having isolated an 'at-risk' mother using this screening policy, our attention is restricted to the exact risk for that individual pregnancy.

At 'at-risk' maternal serum AFP value defines a specific sub-population in which the prevalence of NTDs is significantly greater than in the unscreened population at large. This 'conditional' prevalence is given directly by the individual posterior probability for the patient's observed serum AFP value.

Reassessment of the individual risk from the patient's amniotic fluid AFP value employs this 'conditional' prevalence in the calculation procedure, i.e. the 'information' provided by the serum AFP value is fully utilized. This is only possible under the assumption that the serum and amniotic fluid AFP levels are *independent* measures of risk (Chapter 3, section 3.3), a reasonable assumption for this situation (Report, 1979).

For the assessment of individual mothers we require individual risk assessments. Screening probabilities have nothing to contribute to the evaluation of individual test results, and they will mislead, particularly for test values in close proximity to the screening cut-off levels.

5A.4

The action to be taken on the basis of these probability assessments is a matter of clinical judgement, balancing the alternative courses of action available against their possible consequences. The desirability of any given consequence can be quantified on a probability scale, the number being referred to as the *utility* of that consequence. The incorporation of utilities (embodying professional value judgements) into the risk assessment program takes us into the field of decision theory, which is beyond the scope of this book. An excellent introduction to the logic and 'arithmetic' of decision theory is provided by Lindley (1978), at quite a modest price.

Remember finally that the use of probabilities in assessing individual cases demands a certain amount of common sense. They are a guide to action—no more, no less. The patient either has condition A or he does not, there is absolutely no uncertainty about that! The uncertainty lies in our ability to correctly divine the true state of affairs obtaining for a particular patient, given the limited information at our disposal.

The procedures described represent an efficient means of clearly representing those uncertainties.

REFERENCES
Second Report of the UK Collaborative Study on Alphafetoprotein in relation to Neural Tube Defects (1979) *Lancet* 2, 651–662.
Lindley D. (1978) *Making Decisions*. New York, Wiley.

6 Quality Control

6.1. INTRODUCTION

If the discipline of statistics has one really essential piece of wisdom to impart to the laboratory analyst, it might be this: that a clinical measurement x is, in isolation, absolutely worthless. It is a little like pointing out to a stranger his position on a map from which all physical and political boundaries have been obliterated. It tells him vaguely where he is but not enough to keep him out of trouble. The boundaries for a laboratory measurement take the form $x \pm y$ where y is an explicitly defined statement of the probable measurement error. If y is small relative to x then we might have rather more confidence in taking action on the value of x than if y were large.

A blood glucose of 10·2 mmol/l $\pm$ 0·2 mmol/l (the interval so defined having a 95% probability of encompassing the 'actual' glucose concentration) is clearly more informative than one of 10·2 mmol/l $\pm$ 2 mmol/l, and both reports are a good deal more informative than the summary report 10·2 mmol/l full-stop, which tells us very little at all. By strict convention, reporting the result to one decimal place implies that the assay method can reliably distinguish 10·2 from 10·1 and 10·3. This implies a random error of considerably less than 1% (the standard deviation would need to be approximately 0·04 mmol/l for the distinction to hold reliably in 95% of the results reported!). If the report of 10·2 was the level of thyroid stimulating hormone in mmol/l as estimated by a radioimmunoassay, a random error of 15% might be quite realistic leaving us with a case of decimal overkill.

In order to qualify measurements in a realistic manner we need some insight into the properties and magnitude of the error term y, which contains all the really useful information about x.

6.2. INACCURACY AND IMPRECISION

Repeated measurements on a single sample reveal two major classes of measurement error: 1. *Systematic bias* or *Inaccuracy*; and 2. *Random error* or *Imprecision*.

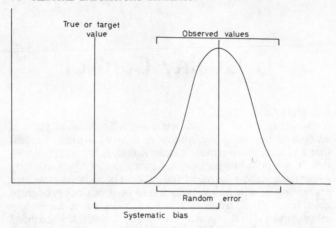

Fig. 26. The basic components of measurement error.

1. *Inaccuracy* may be defined as the difference between the mean of a set of repeated measurements on a particular sample and its 'true' or 'target' value. The true value for complex biological samples cannot be unequivocally determined in an absolute gravimetric sense; the term target value implies a consensus of (expert) opinion as to what constitutes the best *estimate* of the true value, e.g. the result of a definitive assay method.

Systematic bias may arise from fundamental defects in the calibration assumptions. For example, the standard material might not behave in an identical manner to the test material in the assay system. Alternatively bias may arise from transient failures in calibration attributable to instability in the assay conditions (e.g. instrumental drift) or the deterioration of otherwise satisfactory standards (e.g. bacterial contamination).

The former problem is not at all easy to detect or deal with when the assay concerned involves an ill-defined or heterogeneous analyte such as proteins or polypeptide hormones. The problem is considered further in the context of method comparison studies (see Chapter 10). Transient bias or drift is taken up later in this chapter.

2. *Imprecision* is the variability or scatter of repeated measurements about their observed means. *Fig. 26* illustrates the two types of error.

For the majority of assays the random error is the sum of a wide variety of probabilistic elements in the assay procedure, e.g. instrumental variations and fluctuations, a degree of unpredictability in the chemical or biological reaction mechanism and contributions from the analyst and the environment. The number and independence of these factors provide good theoretical grounds for believing that the overall random error distribution might be Normal, and for the raw response data (such as optical density) from a large number of assays this proves to be the case. The way that the raw data is subsequently manipulated by the analyst to obtain his 'result' will affect the error distribution. For example, if the optical densities are translated into concentrations using a non-linear calibration line as in *Fig. 27*, the Normal error distributions of the raw data will be transformed into skewed error distributions for the calculated concentrations. When the uncertainty in the calibration-line itself is taken into account we find that the error-distribution for the estimated concentrations becomes asymmetric *even* with straight-line calibrations. This problem is considered in detail in section 8.7.

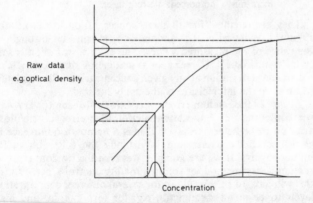

Fig. 27. Relating the random error distribution of the response (raw data) to that of the calculated dose (concentration).

The next problem that arises in considering the error distributions is their relation to the concentration value. In *Fig. 28* a standard curve (or calibration line) is illustrated in which each of the three standards used has been repeatedly assayed in order to gain some insight into the behaviour of the random error distributions as the concentration increases.

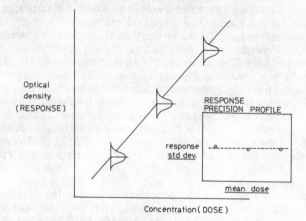

Fig. 28. Random error distributions uniform throughout the measurement range (homoscedastic response).

They are identical for all three concentration levels, i.e. the standard deviation of the random error is constant throughout the range of the measured values. The error distribution is said to be homoscedastic (Greek: equal scatter). A single estimate of the standard deviation at any given concentration will completely summarize the imprecision of the assay method.

In *Fig. 29* the random error distributions are seen to vary with the concentration of the test material. The error distributions are said to be heteroscedastic. This is a common occurrence in clinical chemical assays and is virtually the rule with radio-immunoassays. If we are going to describe the random error of such an assay method, or set up a quality control scheme for it, this will have to be carried out for several different concentration levels to be at all meaningful, e.g. for low, normal and high concentration values.

One exception to this rule is the case where the standard deviation increases as a fixed percentage of the concentration value. In these cases the imprecision of the assay method might be conveniently summarized as a coefficient of variation (c.v.), which is simply the standard deviation expressed as a percentage of its associated mean.

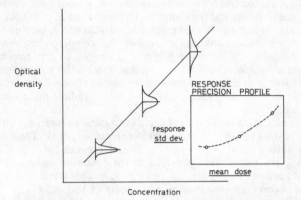

Concentration

Fig. 29. Random error distributions non-uniform throughout the measurement range (heteroscedastic response).

Mean	Std. dev.	c.v.
10	1	10%
100	10	10%
200	20	10%

There are always risks in interpreting quantities that have been transformed out of their original scales of measurement, and the c.v. is no exception. Its use in the context of methodological error cannot be justified until the random error has been firmly established as a percentage function of the concentration. Life being what it is, the relationship between the standard deviation and the concentration is often quite complicated, particularly for immunochemical assay (RIA, EMIT etc.).

The pattern of the random error in any particular assay should be made the subject of a specific pilot study prior to setting up a quality control scheme, in order to determine how much and what sort of control the assay requires.

The imprecision of an assay can be informatively summarized in the form of precision profiles for both the response variable (e.g. optical density) and the dose variable (e.g. concentration).

The imprecision of the assay (standard deviation) is determined on the response and the estimated concentration at a number of points throughout the range of clinical interest. A plot of the *response* standard deviation against the corresponding mean responses on a simple x–y graph gives rise to the *response precision profile*. This is often quite characteristic for a given assay and forms an important preliminary step in the optimization of immunochemical assays, in particular radioimmunoassays (Ekins, 1977).

A plot of the *dose* standard deviation against the corresponding mean dose values gives rise to the *dose precision profile*. These can be differentiated into within-batch and between-batch profiles using the information provided in the following section (6.3). They are an invaluable aid in estimating, by simple interpolation, the uncertainty associated with a variety of text values.

The standard deviation at zero dose $\times$ 2·6 represents the minimum amount of analyte that can be distinguished from baseline 'noise" with 95 % certainty.

6.3. WITHIN-BATCH AND BETWEEN-BATCH IMPRECISION

The factors contributing to the overall random error of an assay have been briefly referred to. If we extend our consideration of the assay to its behaviour over a period of days, weeks or months, then a number of additional sources of variation will be introduced into the picture, e.g. different analysts, different (or deteriorating) reagents, changing environmental conditions etc., all of which will inflate the long-term variation.

W. S. Gosset, writing under his statistical pseudonym 'Student' (1917) made the following comments on the subject which are difficult to improve upon:

'After considerable experience I have not encountered any determination which is not influenced by the date on which it is made; from this it follows that a number of determinations of the same thing made on the same day are likely to lie more closely together than if the repetitions had been made on different days.'

The case for describing measurement random error at two levels, within-batch and between-batch, seems to be clear.

The classical approach to this problem has been to assay a

control sample twenty or more times, all in the same batch, and then to assay it in twenty or more consecutive batches. The standard deviations calculated on the two groups of results provide some information on the within-batch and between-batch variations respectively. The primary drawback to this approach is that it tells us only what the variation was like at the time the assays were performed. If the variation was fairly consistent for any given assay the standard deviations might suffice to describe the variation in all subsequent measurements. Unfortunately, for the majority of assays the random error is constantly changing and the nature and magnitude of those changes can often provide valuable insights into the behaviour of the assay. In order to keep our information about the imprecision up to date it would appear that twenty or more replicate assays are going to be required with every assay batch; this is hardly a very realistic proposition for the average hospital laboratory!

The following quality control scheme was described by Rodbard (1974) and its simplicity and economy of design recommend it for consideration.

An appropriate control sample is assayed twice in every batch of test samples, once at the beginning (x_1) and once at the end (x_2) of the batch so as to pick up the maximum effect of instrumental, reagent and analyst fatigue. After ten such pairs of control values have been accumulated the quality control programme can be initiated. The calculations are shown in full in *Table 8*.

Table 8. Quality control data for Human Placental Lactogen assay

Assay	X_1	X_2	$\overline{X_i}$	S_i^2
1	5·0	5·0	5·0	0·00
2	4·8	5·0	4·9	0·02
3	4·8	4·6	4·7	0·02
4	4·6	5·2	4·9	0·18
5	5·1	5·1	5·1	0·00
6	5·1	5·2	5·15	0·005
7	5·0	5·0	5·0	0·00
8	4·6	4·6	4·6	0·00
9	4·5	4·7	4·6	0·02
10	4·6	4·8	4·7	0·02

Note: S_t^2 calculated for each data pair as: $S_t^2 = [(|x_1 - x_2|)/\sqrt{2}]^2$

$$\Sigma \bar{x}_t = 48 \cdot 65$$
$$\Sigma \bar{x}_t^2 = 237 \cdot 05$$
$$\Sigma S_t^2 = 0 \cdot 265$$

Calculate
$$S_{\bar{x}}^2 = [\Sigma \bar{x}^2 - ((\Sigma \bar{x})^2/n)]/(n-1) = [237 \cdot 05 - ((48 \cdot 65)^2/10)]/9$$
$$= 0 \cdot 0411$$

from which:

within-batch standard deviation,
$$S_w = \sqrt{(\Sigma S_t^2/n)} = \sqrt{(0 \cdot 265/10)}$$
$$= 0 \cdot 163$$

Between-batch standard deviation,
$$S_b = \sqrt{[(S_{\bar{x}}^2 - S_w^2/2) + S_w^2]}$$
$$= \sqrt{[0 \cdot 0411 - (0 \cdot 163)^2/2) + (0 \cdot 163)^2]}$$
$$= 0 \cdot 233.$$

The within-batch standard deviation, S_w, and the between-batch standard deviation, S_b, can be updated with every new batch of acceptable results by adding on the latest values for x_1 and x_2 and discarding the oldest two values.

The S_w is obtained by pooling ten individual variance estimates (each based on two results). Individually these variances are of dubious value, but pooled they convey a good deal of useful information. The pooling does result in some loss of sensitivity to changes in precision but this is a small price to pay given the alternative of heavy replication in every assay batch.

The S_b is somewhat less straightforward in calculation since we have to disentangle the two sources of error in this very compact design. The calculations are an application of the technique known as the Analysis of Variance, or ANOVA for short.

Rodbard discusses in some detail the applications of the S_w and S_b for the quality control of radioimmunoassays, and the calculations involved when the control samples are assayed more than twice in each batch.

6.4. USING THE S_w AND S_b

1. An immediate application of the S_w is in bringing the concept of $x \pm y$ to life. If we are correct in assuming a Normal distribution for the random error we can be approximately 95% certain that the estimated test concentration $\pm 2 S_w$ encompasses the 'target' concentration of the material being measured. The

assay method used should be quoted on the report along with the appropriate clinical reference intervals as established by that same method. The validity of this interpretation rests very heavily on the assumption that the control sample(s) behave in every respect like the test samples. This is a technical problem rather than a statistical one.

Pools of low, medium and high concentration human test samples are probably the best source of control material, providing that they are rigorously checked for health hazards such as Australia antigen. Citrated plasma from time expired blood transfusion units and animal sera must be regarded with caution. It is impossible to establish beyond doubt that these materials behave in every respect like human serum; indeed it is almost certain that they do not.

2. The statistics S_w and S_b have a potentially valuable role to play in the interpretation of changes in serial assays on the same patient. Consider the assay of a material such as human placental lactogen (HPL), where the change in concentration from one sample to the next may be of considerable importance in assessing placental function during the third trimester of pregnancy.

The current HPL assay quality control statistics are:

$$\text{Control sample mean} = 5 \cdot 0 \quad \text{mg/l},$$
$$S_w = 0 \cdot 10 \text{ mg/l},$$
$$S_b = 0 \cdot 23 \text{ mg/l}.$$

Imagine that we have two samples of serum from a patient taken on consecutive days and assayed in *separate* batches:

Results: Serum 1 = 5·4 mg/l,
Serum 2 = 5·0 mg/l.

We want to know whether the apparent fall in HPL concentration reflects a genuine change or is simply random error, i.e. if the two samples had identical 'true' HPL values is it likely that the measured values could exhibit a variation as great as that observed.

Since we are dealing with between-batch variation we need to call upon S_b to assess the statistical significance of the difference in the observed values. From the ongoing QC programme we find this to be 0·23 mg/l.

The test statistic required can be reduced to the following very simple procedure.

Test statistic = (Highest assay value − Lowest assay value)/S_b
$$= (5\cdot4 - 5\cdot0)/0\cdot23 = 1\cdot74.$$

The 95% critical value for this test is 2·77 and the 99% critical value, 3·63. The derivation of these two values is relatively straightforward using tables of the Normal probability integral (1). Since the test statistic of 1·74 is less than the 95% critical value of 2·77 we conclude that there is a greater than 1:20 chance of such a difference being observed with samples actually having the same underlying 'true' values, i.e. the observed fall in HPL concentration, may very well be due to nothing more than measurement error.

Reconsider these two results as if they were obtained from the *same* batch of assays. We are now dealing with within-batch variation only, the statistic required being the S_w. This is currently 0·1 mg/l.

$$\text{Test statistic} = (5\cdot4 - 5\cdot0)/0\cdot10 = 4\cdot00.$$

Since the test statistic is greater than 3·63, there is less than a 1:100 chance that such a difference in the measured HPL values could have arisen with samples having the same underlying 'true' values, i.e. it is highly likely that the observed fall in HPL values reflect a genuine physiological change.

A number of important points are made by this simple exercise. *No* scientific interpretation of the apparent change in HPL values could have been made at all without up-to-date information on the within-batch and between-batch variation of the assay.

The analysis is only valid if the patient's test values are in the same concentration range as the control serum used to establish the S_w and S_b values. This is because the random error associated with the HPL radioimmunoassay is heteroscedastic; it varies with the concentration. Standard deviations calculated on the results from a control sample of 3·0 g/l have *no* relevance whatsoever to the imprecision of a test sample of 10·0 g/l.

6.4.1. Analytical goals

Competing interests demand assays that are cheap, accurate, reproducible, fast and available 24 hours a day. Keeping everyone happy has, in the past, owed rather more to serendipity than science (assuming for one moment that they are all happy!). This situation will change given the sums of money involved in the laboratory aspect of health care.

The definition of analytical goals first requires a clear and unambiguous statement of the clinical requirements. By way of example, suppose that the clinical staff demand an assay for maternal serum HPL that can detect a change of 0·4 mg/l from one assay batch to the next. What sort of precision should the laboratory be aiming for to satisfy this requirement? Reference to section 6·4 suggests that the necessary between-batch S_b is $(0·4 \text{ mg/l})/2·77 = 0·14$ mg/l, which will satisfy the clinical requirement 95% of the time.

The clinical demand has been effectively translated into laboratory practice, but life is not as simple as the example suggests. Problems abound. We already know that analytical imprecision is, in most cases, concentration dependent. The clinician may have to specify the concentration range within which his requirements are to be satisfied.

The analyte considered may exhibit a degree of quite natural variation within any given subject, during the course of a day and from one day to the next. This *biological variation* is quite distinct from the variability associated with our observation (measurement) process and must influence the interpretation given to observed changes in analyte concentration.

What happens when we come to consider serial assay values (three or more on one patient)? Relatively small changes, a lot less than the critical 2·77 S_b, all in the same general direction, may constitute a significant *trend*, suggesting the need for a more detailed retrospective analysis of the laboratory reports.

The problems in this area were addressed by the Aspen Conference on Analytical Goals in Clinical Chemistry in 1976 (Elevitch, 1977). The statistical aspects of analytical goal-setting are discussed by Harris (1979).

6.4.2. Accepting or rejecting the results of an assay

One of the objectives of a quality control programme must be to signal to the analyst that he is not meeting defined criteria for an acceptable assay. So far we have treated the S_w and S_b values as mirrors, reflecting the precision status of the assay. Translating this information into effective criteria for accepting or rejecting the results of a particular assay batch requires some careful thought.

Graphical methods have been widely employed to set limits on acceptable drift or imprecision. A control sample is assayed repeatedly over a period of time during which the assay method is judged to be performing satisfactorily, e.g. from inter-method and inter-laboratory comparison studies. The mean and standard deviation of the estimated control values are used in the construction of a simple control chart, illustrated in *Fig. 30*, the assumption of a Normal distribution for the analytical random errors being implicit. The control sample is subsequently assayed in parallel with test samples (its identity as a control sample being concealed), the value obtained being plotted on the control chart above the assay date. As long as the control values fluctuate about the control mean with no more than 5% of the recorded values outside of the $\pm 2S$ limits, all is judged to be well according to the received wisdom! More than 5% of the control values outside the $2S$ limits suggests deteriorating precision and values outside of the $3S$ limits would constitute grounds for rejection of the assay batch concerned, such a value being expected only once in every hundred control analyses.

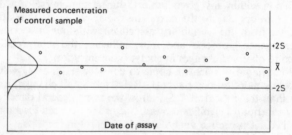

Fig. 30. Simple Shewhart quality control chart.

For many assay methods the S_b is sufficiently stable in time to permit the construction of such a chart, adjustments to the control limits being made as necessary to accommodate accumulating information about the control sample itself, and to reflect changes in the analytical methodology or instrumentation.

For many other assays the imprecision fluctuates to such an extent (*see* the TSH assay data in *Table 9*) that it is difficult to see how such a control chart could reasonably be maintained, or for that matter logically justified. The continual readjustment of the control limits might prove rather more trouble than it was worth. If the analyst does not get more *out* of his quality control programme than he puts *in*, he will soon find plausible reasons for letting it slip into disuse.

Table 9. Within-batch (S_w) and between-batch (S_b) variation for two assays, one quite precise (T_3) and the other relatively imprecise (TSH)

	Assay		
T_3 uptake %		TSH mu/l	
S_w	S_b	S_w	S_b
1·72	2·24	0·68	1·05
1·77	1·94	0·59	1·39
1·83	2·02	0·62	1·39
1·84	1·98	0·61	1·42
1·80	2·00	0·65	1·18
1·80	2·00	0·77	1·73
1·22	1·69	0·65	1·74
1·16	1·58	1·19	1·85
0·95	1·60	1·23	2·04
1·02	1·42	1·22	2·00
Control mean = 103%		Control mean = 11 mu/L	

Note: TSH = thyroid stimulating hormone; mu/l = milliunits per litre.

The simple control chart described above is widely employed as a basis for 'quality control' but it cannot of itself define the 'quality' that it is supposed to be controlling. What the imprecision of the assay method was yesterday is not, in isolation, a very logical basis for defining the permissible imprecision of the assay method tomorrow! Only the laboratory manager can define the 'quality' required in his laboratory's output, this being a considered synthesis of local clinical expectations (section 6.4.1) and prevailing technical and economic realities. In theory there is no limit to the precision that can be achieved by an assay method: in practice the pursuit of unnecessary precision is, as observed by Aristotle, the mark of uneducated men.

Clinical target values should be defined locally for every laboratory, in terms of the maximum acceptable S_w and S_b

values for each assay method. These can be updated with advances in available technology. The estimated S_w and S_b values from the quality control programme are maintained for use in the daily decision-making process, but the clinical target values provide objective limits beyond which the assay methods are failing to deliver an effective clinical service, in terms of the locally available resources.

A further weakness of the simple control-chart is its insensitivity to low-level drift, i.e. a shift in the accuracy base of the assay method. *Fig. 31* presents a set of control sample values, (*a*) on a simple control chart and (*b*) on a cumulative sum or *cusum* chart, the preparation of which is illustrated in *Table 10*. Although the shift away from the control mean is evident on the simple control chart, it is easy to overlook, the more so given an element of psychological reassurance from the containment of the control values within the $\pm 2S_b$ limits. The evidence of the *cusum* chart simply cannot be ignored.

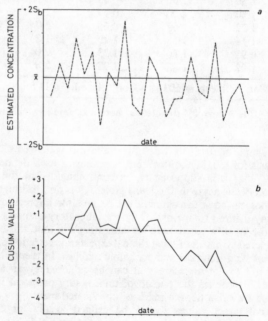

Fig. 31. Comparison of Shewhart (*a*) and cusum (*b*) charts.

Table 10. Control mean $(\bar{X}) = 5 \cdot 0$ mg/l

Assay date	Observed control value X_i	$X_i - \bar{X}$	Cusum value $\Sigma(X_i - \bar{X})$
1	5·0	0·0	0·0
2	4·8	−0·2	−0·2
3	4·8	−0·2	−0·4
4	4·6	−0·4	−0·8
5	5·1	+0·1	−0·7
6	5·1	+0·1	−0·6
7	5·0	0·0	−0·6
8	4·6	−0·4	−1·0
9	4·5	−0·5	−1·5
10	4·6	−0·4	−1·9

The cusum chart tells us very little about the imprecision of the assay but a great deal about changes in the accuracy base. The method is heavily dependent upon the validity of the control sample mean as an estimate of the 'true value' with respect to that assay method; it is worth spending some time getting this right. The cusum method has its roots in manufacturing industry where the 'control mean' was a production target defined by the manufacturer, e.g. $1 \cdot 5$ cm nails. In the clinical laboratory the control mean cannot be 'defined'; it has to be estimated in the face of analytical error.

As a general rule of thumb, any sustained movement of the cusum data line away from the control mean line is a cause for concern: the sharper the angle of the departure, the more severe the bias involved. The slope of the line is dependent on the scaling of the chart. When single control values are being recorded a useful rule for scaling is to set one horizontal unit equal to $2S_b$ vertical units, where S_b is the between-batch standard deviation. A control value that is $2S_b$ away from the control mean will, on this scaling, result in a cusum value at 45° to the horizontal, relative to the last plotted cusum point. Objective assessment of the cusum chart is possible using a V-mask, the procedure being illustrated in *Fig. 32*. A plastic or Perspex mask is placed over the chart with the point of the V located at a distance d ahead of the last plotted cusum point. If all of the previously plotted points fall within the angle of the V, the assay method is judged to be in control.

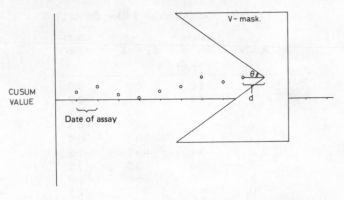

Fig. 32. Decision making V-mask for the cusum control chart.

The angle of the V is 2θ. The choice of values for d and θ determines the degree of control exercised. The smaller these two values are, the smaller the drift that is required for rejection to occur. If the scaling is standardized as described, tables of values for d and θ are available to meet the analyst's requirements (Woodward and Goldsmith, 1964). As previously indicated, the S_b for many assays is itself somewhat variable, necessitating a more subjective assessment of the cusum chart. If the chart is sensibly scaled, the control mean realistic and the bias worth worrying about, it will be difficult to ignore the divergent cusum line. More than five cusum points in a trend away from the control mean line is a cause for concern.

The following criteria for accepting or rejecting the results of an assay are suggestions only. Ultimately the degree of control you want is the control you will get! It is assumed that three control samples, reflecting three different concentration levels, are assayed twice in each test batch, the identity of the control materials being disguised as far as is possible.

1. *Within-batch precision control*

If the difference between any one of the control duplicates exceeds $3 \cdot 63 \, S_w$, reject the assay.

If the difference between any two of the control duplicates exceeds $2 \cdot 77 S_w$, reject the assay. One control pair in excess of this value would be grounds for caution in assessing the assay batch.

2. *Between-batch precision control*

If any *single* control estimate falls outside the range of the control mean $\pm\ 3S_b$, reject the assay.

If any two control estimates fall outside the range of the control mean $\pm\ 2S_b$, reject the assay. One control value outside this range should be noted since it is not expected to happen more than once with every 20 control estimates (approximately).

3. *Within-batch drift control*

Calculate the mean of each of the three control duplicates. Two duplicate means both in excess of the control mean $+2(S_w/\sqrt{2})$ *or* both less than the control mean $-2(S_w/\sqrt{2})$, suggest a loss of calibration control.

All three of the duplicate means in excess of the control mean $+1(S_w/\sqrt{2})$ *or* all less than the control mean $-1(S_w/\sqrt{2})$, suggest a loss of calibration control

4. *Between-batch drift control*

Use the control duplicate means to prepare and update the cusum charts. This will require the scaling to be modified such that one horizontal unit is set equal to $2S_b/\sqrt{n}$ vertical units, where $n = 2$. Check the updated cusum charts for evidence of practically significant drift.

Borderline assessments must take into account the information available from supplementary controls, patient replicates and calibration data.

The results obtained on patient's samples carried over from one test batch to the next as a check on reproducibility should agree within $2 \cdot 77\ S_b$ (95% of the time).

The results obtained on commercially prepared control materials should be within $\pm\ 2S_w$ of the target value for the methodology employed, assuming that the general reliability of the material used has been satisfactorily assessed.

If the assay batch is accepted, the quality control programme is updated with the latest set of control estimates. If the re-calculated S_w and S_b values (based on the latest 10 pairs of control estimates for each control level), are within the clinical target values for these quantities, the patients' test values can be released.

If an executive decision is taken to release test data associated with borderline control values, the quality control programme *must* be updated with that control data set. If, as a result of this action, the re-estimated S_w and S_b values are in excess of the clinical target values, the override decision should be reversed, the control programme reset to its original status and the test samples re-assayed. The control programme should at all times reflect the quality of the test values actually released to the clinical staff.

An excellent overview of the accuracy of the assay method can be obtained from participation in local or national inter-laboratory quality control schemes. It is difficult to sustain an argument that you are right and everyone else is wrong (with the exception of some polypeptide hormone assays in which 'right' poses a number of slippery philosophical problems). The information supplied from external quality control schemes may arrive 2 weeks after the event, but it is certainly better to know you are hopelessly out of line with the national consensus 2 weeks late than never at all!

6.5. PATIENT BASED PRECISION STUDIES

In a small laboratory there may be practical difficulties in implementing a control scheme in which the identity of the control materials can be effectively concealed over an extended period of time. The colour, opacity or even the viscosity of the control material may identify it in a small assay batch. Even with the best will in the world bias can creep into the treatment of known control samples. There is some irony in the observation that the conscientious analyst will tire more as a result of his sustained concentration than will his careless colleague, making him more susceptible to the effects of unconscious bias.

The estimated imprecision of the analytical method must be based on a completely random sampling of the assay's performance if it is to reflect adequately the uncertainties associated with patients' test values.

Patient based replicates provide an excellent basis for achieving this objective. An assayed test sample is harvested from the day's workload, stored overnight under suitable conditions, and re-introduced into the next day's analytical run under an assumed name, taking care to avoid confusion with existing patients. After ten such samples have been assayed in duplicate, the between-batch imprecision of the assay method can be estimated as follows:

	First result X_1	Second result X_2	S_i^2
1	109	114	12·5
2	93	90	4·5
3	44	48	8·0
4	192	171	220·5
5	31	32	0·5
6	64	69	12·5
7	101	114	84·5
8	140	147	24·5
9	74	74	0·0
10	78	91	84·5

where (ignoring sign)

$$S_i^2 = [|X_1 - X_2|/\sqrt{2}]^2$$

$$\Sigma S_i^2 = 452\cdot0$$

$$S_w = \sqrt{(\Sigma S_i^2/n)}$$

$$= \sqrt{(452/10)} = 6\cdot72$$

An estimate of the within-batch S_w could be obtained by splitting samples for duplicate analysis within the same batch. The analysis of the data would be identical to that above. With every new pair of sample values, the analysis can be updated using the latest ten pairs of values. The patient based scheme provides absolutely no information at all about the accuracy of the assay. Properly conducted, it provides excellent information regarding its imprecision.

6.6 PATIENTS' DAILY MEANS

Calculation of the overall mean of all the test samples assayed in a particular day or batch has been described as a valuable supplementary control procedure in the clinical laboratory. Most analysts are familiar with the experience of 'low' days or 'high' days, when there appears to have been a general shift in the level of results observed. Sometimes this is obvious: often it is a less tangible, almost a subjective feeling. The calculation of daily or batch means formalizes the observation of such shifts.

In practice it is necessary to truncate or trim the test sample values such that extreme values (low or high) are excluded from consideration. The truncation limits are not objectively defined and need to be estimated locally in the light of the prevailing population characteristics from which the laboratory draws its workload. The interpretation of changes in the daily mean and its use as a basis for action (accepting or rejecting assay batches) is also a matter for the individual laboratory. Simple in principle, the method does demand a good deal of homework in application if it is to prove an effective aid in the decision-making process. The interested reader is referred to Whitehead (1977) for a clear discussion of the problems.

A major criticism of the daily or batch mean concerns its sensitivity to non-random sampling patterns in the specimen intake. For example, a specialist clinic may account for a substantial proportion of the specimens received by the laboratory on a particular day, shifting the daily mean for purely non-technical reasons.

The problem can be tackled by employing a moving-average in place of the simple arithmetic mean. This is a technique employed in the analysis of time-series, e.g. economic trends, for separating out the trend (signal) from seasonal or biological fluctuations (noise). In its simplest form, a proportion of the previous day's data is carried over into the calculation of the new day's mean, thereby smoothing-out irregularities.

Today's Moving Average, $MA_t = q \cdot \bar{X}_t + ((1 - q) \cdot MA_{t-1})$

where MA_{t-1} is the previous day's moving average,

$\bar{X}_t$ is today's arithmetic mean,

and q is the smoothing factor taking values between 0 and 1.

For example, suppose we set the smoothing factor q at 0.4 with $MA_{t-1} = 110$ and today's $\bar{X}_t = 119$:

$MA_t = (0.4 \times 119) + ((1 - 0.4) \cdot 110) = 113.6$.

If this procedure is combined with a truncation procedure to exclude extreme analyte values it becomes a robust yet sensitive indicator of systematic bias. The smoothing factor appropriate to any particular assay is a matter of local experiment.

These ideas have been extended by Bull et al. (1974) for application to the quality control of haematology investigations employing automated analyzers; in particular, to monitor the calibration stability of such equipment. The erythrocyte indices, Mean Corpuscular Haemoglobin (MCH), Mean Corpuscular Haemoglobin Concentration (MCHC) and Mean Corpuscular Volume (MCV) were selected in view of the relative stability of their mean values in healthy populations. The use of a patient based control system has particular appeal in the haematologic context given the technical problems involved in providing control materials for cell counts of assured long-term stability.

6.7. COUNTING ERRORS

The errors associated with counting procedures in the medical laboratory generally exhibit a Poisson distribution. This probability distribution is characteristically associated with the observation of completely *random* events in a continuum such as space or time. It can be considered as a particular case of the binomial distribution (expression 4.1) in which the probability (p) of the event of interest is very small and the number of trials (n) is infinite. Under these restrictions it makes sense to ask how many times the event occurs, e.g. how many reticulocytes are there in a square millimetre of blood film, but it makes *no* sense at all to ask how many times the event does not occur! You might contrast this with a typical binomial experiment.

A unique feature of the Poisson distribution is the numerical equivalence of its mean and variance. This property can be used to check the assumption of randomness. For example, if the observed mean and variance of repeated counts on a well-mixed bacterial suspension differ by more than would be expected from sampling variation alone we would have good grounds for reconsidering the behaviour of the bacterial cells in the suspension. If the variance were greater than the mean it would suggest that the bacteria were *aggregating* or clumping. Alternatively, if the variance were less than the mean it would indicate some regularity in the dispersion of the bacterial cells, possibly due to mutual *repulsion*. The probability distributions generated in these non-random situations have considerable importance in the treatment of stochastic processes (Chapter 3) particularly in biology and economics.

Since the mean of the Poisson distribution is numerically identical to its variance (or standard deviation squared), the relative error of a counting process will decrease as the size of the count increases. It is as well to be clear what this means. Imagine that we have recorded the number of radioactive emissions from a test sample in a 4-second interval and a 400-second interval. The observed counts, their standard deviation $[S = \sqrt{(count)}]$ and coefficients of variation [c.v. $= (S/\text{count} \times 100]$ are reported in *Table 11*.

Table 11

Time	Count	S	c.v.
4 s	100	10	10%
400 s	10 000	100	1%

The *relative* counting error (c.v.) goes down as the count increases, *but* the *absolute* error (S) goes up. It is commonly stated that the absolute error of a count (isotopic, bacteriological or haematological) is reduced by increasing the number of counts recorded. This is strictly true only in considering the rate of the count per unit time (or volume for cell counts), i.e. suppose that the object of *Table 11* was the calculation of the rate of counts/second.

Using the *4s count* we have:

Mean counts/s	$= 100/4$	$= 25$ counts/s,
Variance	$= 100/(4)^2$	$= 6\cdot25$,
S	$= \sqrt{6\cdot25}$	$= 2\cdot5$ counts/s.

Using the *400s count* we have:

Mean counts/s	$= 10\,000/400$	$= 25$ counts/s,
Variance	$= 10\,000/(400)^2$	$= 0\cdot0625$
S	$= \sqrt{0\cdot0625}$	$= 0\cdot25$ counts/s.

The estimated rate from the 400s count is considerably more precise than the estimate obtained from the 4s count. This is a rather reassuring confirmation of what common-sense might lead us to expect.

REFERENCES

Bull B. S., Elashoff R.M., Heilbron D.C. et al. (1974) A study of various estimators for the derivation of Quality Control procedures from patient erythrocyte indices. *Am. J. Clin. Pathol.* **61**, 473–481.

Ekins R. P. (1977) *Quality control and assay design* In: *Radioimmunoassay and related Procedures in Medicine.* Vol 2. Vienna, IAEA.

Elevitch F. R. ed. (1977) *Proceedings of the 1976 Aspen Conference on Analytical Goals in Clinical Chemistry*. Skokie, Ill., College of American Pathologists.

Harris E. K. (1979) Statistical principles underlying analytic goal-setting in clinical chemistry. *Am. J. Clin. Pathol.* **72**, 374–382.

Pearson E. S. (1942) The probability integral of the range in samples of n observations from a normal population. *Biometrika* **32**, 302–307.

Rodbard D. (1974) Statistical quality control and routine data processing for radioimmunoassays and immunoradiometric assays. *Clin. Chem.* **20**, 1255–1270.

Whitehead T. P. (1977) *Quality Control in Clinical Chemistry*. New York, Wiley.

Woodward R. H. and Goldsmith T. L. *Cumulative Sum Techniques*. ICI Monograph No 3. (1964) Edinburgh and London, Oliver and Boyd.

7 Inference

Joyous distrust is a sign of health. Everything absolute belongs to pathology. Nietzsche.

A common complaint against the subject of statistics is that there are so many different symbols for the 'same thing'. It is usually the subject of inference that initiates this remark. The symbolism is necessary but by no means standardized. Before tackling any textbook or paper with a statistical content, get acquainted with the author's choice of notation.

7.1. POPULATIONS AND SAMPLES

We define a population as any fully specified group of variables in which we have a particular interest. It may be quite literally the population of a country or a town, or it may be the population of vaccine ampoules of a particular batch number produced by a specific firm in January! It may be the population of throws of a particular dice which is, on the face of it, infinite! All that is really important is that our population be clearly defined.

In the majority of practical situations it would be a formidable task to collect the information we require on every member of the population, and for an infinite population it would be impossible. In order to obtain an *estimate* of the population properties in which we are interested, we can take a reasonably manageable sample from the population, examine its properties, and use these to infer the properties of the population. For the inference to be valid the sample must be fully *representative* of the population from which it was drawn. It must be obtained by an acceptable random sampling procedure. Badly collected samples have a good deal in common with dead patients: no amount of good treatment will make them any better!

If we want to estimate the incidence of poverty in a certain city and select a convenient 'random' sample using the telephone directory for that city, we will find a remarkable absence of the condition we are looking for. The sample may be as random as they come *but* it is only representative of the listed telephone owners who can, presumably, afford the rental! The example is perhaps trivial but some extraordinary blunders have entered the literature of science from failures to define clearly the population considered and the validity of the samples chosen to represent it. The problems become quite acute in the pharmaceutical sciences where the 'sample' may be caged beagle dogs whilst the 'population' of real interest is human.

We will assume that the population properties we are interested in are the mean and standard deviation. These are referred to as *population parameters* and are denoted by Greek letters as follows:

$$\text{the population mean} = \mu;$$
$$\text{the population standard deviation} = \sigma.$$

The calculated mean and standard deviation of a sample drawn from that population are referred to as sample statistics and are denoted by Arabic letters:

$$\text{the sample mean} = \bar{x};$$
$$\text{the sample standard deviation} = S.$$

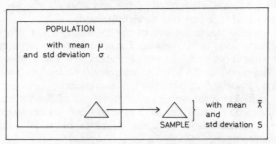

Fig. 33. Population parameters and sample statistics.

When a sample is fully representative of the parent population, the sample statistics are *estimators* of the population parameters (*Fig. 33*). Since they are 'estimates' we do not imagine for a moment that they are identical to the population values. Second and third samples drawn from the same population under similarly controlled conditions will yield further estimates of the parameters that will differ to some extent from each other. The size of the differences that occur is directly related to the size of the samples. If every sample were so big it actually comprised the entire population, the sample statistics would be identical to the population parameters and hence to each other. There would be no sampling variation in the statistics.

The moment that the samples are reduced in size the sample statistics acquire an element of uncertainty as estimates of the parameters, this reaching a maximum when the samples become so small that they comprise just one member of the population. In simple English, the bigger the sample the more reliable the statistics.

7.2. PROPERTIES OF ESTIMATORS
A great deal of mathematical statistics concerns itself with the properties of estimators and in this context a number of words in common use assume quite specialized meanings: *consistency; efficiency; unbiasedness; sufficiency*. By way of example, consistency is a property implied in the last paragraph, i.e. the larger the sample becomes the closer the sample statistics $\bar{x}$ and S approach the population parameters μ and σ. Not all estimators exhibit this property and the assessment of problems at this level is very much the province of the specialist for the very good reason that it is far from straightforward.

Figure 34 illustrates two of the most important properties: efficiency and unbiasedness. The distributions represent the sampling variation in the sample statistic ($\bar{x}$). The properties are not unrelated to the ideas of accuracy (unbiasedness) and precision (efficiency) in laboratory measurements.

A sufficient estimator is one that uses *all* of the 'information' in the sample data. The arithmetic mean $\bar{x}$ is a consistent, unbiased, efficient and sufficient estimator of μ. It cannot be improved upon.

The standard deviation S was originally derived as the root mean square deviation of expression 2.4, with the sample size n as a divisor. As such it is a biased estimator of σ. The bias can be simply removed using $n-1$ as a divisor hence the modification in expression 2.5. Some authors use a small s or the symbol $\hat{\sigma}$ to denote that they are using the unbiased sample standard deviation. It rather depends upon whose book you are reading. For our purposes we will stick to a capital S and assume the use of $n-1$.

Although somewhat technical, this aspect of inference is worth a mention as a caution against the indiscriminate use of the terms referred to, or their too literal interpretation in the statistical literature.

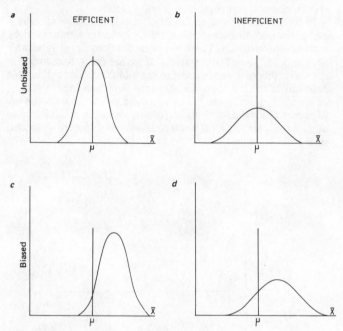

Fig. 34. Some properties of estimators.

7.3. CONFIDENCE INTERVALS

Whenever we employ sample statistics as estimates of population parameters we need to qualify our statements with some indication of their variability. This is greatly facilitated by a curious property of sample statistic distributions.

Suppose that we draw three hundred samples, each of fifty observations, from a single population. If we calculate each of three hundred sample means and look at *their* frequency distribution we will see something not unlike *Fig. 34a.* Appropriate tests would reveal the frequency distribution to be quite compatible with a Normal distribution. What is remarkable about this observation is that it holds for almost all sample statistics, even those calculated from samples that are drawn from non-Normal populations. This appearance of the Normal distribution in the mathematics of sampling distributions confirms its central role in classical statistical theory and practice.

It follows that if the variation of sample statistics such as $\bar{x}$ has a Normal distribution then this is logically summarized by a standard deviation. There are complications here! A sample standard deviation S is a statistic. If we are going to summarize the variability of S we are going to run into the not inconsiderable problem of talking about the standard deviation (or variability) of a standard deviation. We escape the confusion with a change of name. The standard deviation of sample statistics is referred to as a *standard error* (s.e.). The ideas developed so far are illustrated in *Fig. 35*.

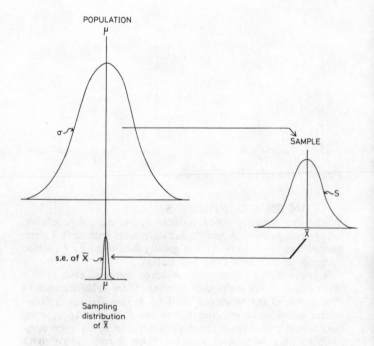

Fig. 35. Sample statistics have their own sampling distributions!

Standard error of the sample mean:

$$\text{s.e. of } \bar{x} = S/\sqrt{n},$$ 7.1

where n = sample size.

If n is greater than 60 the standard error behaves exactly like any other standard deviation, i.e. the $\bar{x} \pm 2(\text{s.e.})$ encompasses 95% of the sampling distribution of $\bar{x}$. A little algebra extends this result so that we can state that there is a 95% probability that $\bar{x} \pm 2(\text{s.e.})$ encompasses μ. We have constructed a 95% *confidence interval* (c.i.) for the population mean! 19 out of 20 such intervals will embrace μ. The sample mean $\bar{x}$ is referred to as a *point estimate* of μ. The 95% c.i. is referred to as an interval estimate on μ. Interval estimates are far more useful in that they convey quite clearly just how much faith we can put in the estimate. A point estimate in isolation is of very little practical use for inference.

Example 7.1

Sample size	=	60.
Sample $\bar{x}$	=	8·0.
Sample S	=	1·580.
s.e. of $\bar{x}$	=	$1·580/\sqrt{60} = 0·20.$
95% c.i.	=	$\bar{x} \pm 2 \text{ (s.e. of } \bar{x})$
	=	$8·0 \pm 0·40$
	=	7·60–8·40.

There is a 95% probability that the interval 7·60–8·40 encompasses the population mean μ. Our *best* estimate of μ is 8·0.

Example 7.2

Sample size	=	5.
Sample $\bar{x}$	=	8·0.
Sample S	=	1·580.
s.e. of $\bar{x}$	=	$1·580/\sqrt{5} = 0·71.$

When the sample size is less than 60 the distribution of the sample statistics becomes rather more 'spread' than would be expected for a Normal distribution, this increasing as the samples get smaller and smaller. The sample statistic exhibits a *t*-distribution, for which a table of integrals is supplied in *Table F* (Appendix). We locate the required value of *t* by reading down the left hand column of *Table F* to $n-1$ (for this example, $n-1 = 4$)

and then reading across to the required probability level, e.g. 5%. *Check* that you are in the correct column by reading down to $n = 60$, which should have a tabulated 5% value of 2·000. In some *t*-tables you will find this located under the 2·5% value, in which case this is the column you should refer to. The reason is taken up later in this chapter under the heading of one-tailed and two-tailed tests. For our example $t_{(0.05)} = 2·78$. Therefore:

$$95\% \text{ c.i. on } \mu = \bar{x} \quad \pm[t_{(0.05)} \times \text{s.e. of } \bar{x}]$$
$$= 8·0 \quad \pm[2·78 \times 0·71]$$
$$= 6·03\text{--}9·97.$$

There is a 95% probability that the interval 6·03–9·97 encompasses the population mean μ. Our best estimate of μ is 8·0. The increased uncertainty of our estimates from the smaller sample is made clear in the interval estimate. Never accept other people's 'statistics' without ascertaining for yourself the uncertainty implicit in them. A computer will quite happily provide you with a point estimate of 8·000 19. Set against a 95% c.i. of 6–10 it is not quite so impressive.

7.4. HYPOTHESIS TESTING

The ideas so briefly introduced about standard errors and confidence intervals are developed to a level of considerable sophistication in the testing of hypotheses. This subject concerns itself with questions of the form: 'Is the difference observed between, for example, two sample means, due to nothing more than their combined sampling variation; or is the difference between them so great that some alternative explanation must be sought?'

We have already encountered a simple hypothesis test in dealing with the sample coefficients of skewness and kurtosis, in Chapter 4. The question posed there was somewhat simpler inasmuch as we were concerned with the difference between a sample coefficient and a *fixed* value (the 'expected' value for a Normal distribution). Was the difference observed a consequence of sampling variation alone, or did it reflect a real deviation from Normality in the underlying population?

Example 7.3

To illustrate some of the thinking behind the *hypothesis test* (or *significance test*) we will return to *Example 7.2*. Suppose that we had some grounds for believing that the sample (of 5 observations) had come from a particular population whose mean μ_0 is known to be exactly 7·000. Is it likely that a random sample of five observations drawn from this population will have a sample mean of 8·000?

For the hypothesis test this question is framed in a rather formal way. We propose a *null hypothesis* H_0: that the mean of the population μ_1, from which the sample was drawn, is identical to that of the reference population whose mean we know to be $\mu_0 = 7·000$.

$$H_0: \mu_1 = \mu_0$$

Next we require an *alternative hypothesis* H_1: μ_1 is not equal to μ_0. This is generally the more important hypothesis from a practical point of view:

$$H_1: \mu_1 \neq \mu_0$$

This may appear rather elaborate, but it is important. In order to determine the likely truth or otherwise of H_1 we require a *test statistic*. This is a property of the sample data that behaves differently when H_1 is true, from when H_1 is untrue. The test statistic must have a *critical value*. If the test statistic falls short of the critical value we conclude that there is insufficient evidence for rejecting H_0 in favour of H_1. *Note this wording carefully. We* can *never* prove that H_0 is *true*. We simply fail to provide evidence that it it is not true. This is not as absurd as it sounds, but is quite in line with contemporary scientific philosophy.

If the test statistic exceeds the critical value we reject H_0 in favour of H_1. The evidence of the sample, as embodied in the test statistic, suggests that H_0 is unlikely to be true.

The critical region of the test statistic is determined by the significance level of the test.

The *significance level* is the probability we are prepared to accept of being wrong in rejecting H_0 for H_1 on the basis of the test. Probability levels of 5% and 1% have become widely, if arbitrarily, accepted for this purpose. If someone's life depended on the outcome of the test you might prefer considerably less than a 1% chance of being wrong.

For our example problem we require a *t-statistic* and we will accept a 5% *probability* of being wrong in rejecting H_0 for H_1.

$$H_0: \mu_1 = \mu_0$$
$$H_1: \mu_1 \neq \mu_0, \text{ where } \mu_0 = 7 \cdot 0.$$

The truth of the matter is that we have already done all the work that is required. The t-statistic was actually employed in setting up the 95% c.i. for this data. All we have to do is observe whether or not μ_0 (7·0) falls in this interval.

Remember that the 95% c.i. has a 95% probability of encompassing the test population mean μ_1. Since μ_0 does fall in this interval (previously calculated as 6·03–9·97) we conclude that there is a greater than 5% probability that $\mu_1 = 7 \cdot 0$.

Conclusion:

We have insufficient evidence for rejecting the hypothesis $\mu_1 = 7$ in favour of the alternative, $\mu_1 \neq 7 \cdot 0$.

Remember, this does *not* mean that $\mu_1 = 7 \cdot 0$. It simply means that we have failed to produce good evidence that it is not, which is *not* the same thing at all.

The curious will have already noted that our hypothesis test fails to reject H_0 using the small sample of *example 7.2* but *does* reject H_0 in favour of H_1 with the larger sample of *example 7.1*, with the same $\bar{x}$ and S. The 95% c.i. for the larger sample, 7·60–8·40, clearly excludes $\mu_0 = 7 \cdot 0$ at a 5% significance level.

It would appear that all we have to do to obtain a 'significant' result is to employ larger and larger samples until we get the result we want! As the problem has been presented there is some truth in this; what is curious is that this is exactly how the situation is presented in a large number of non-specialist texts. This apparently unscientific conclusion has arisen primarily from failing to specify H_0 in really practical terms. Technology deals with practicalities not absolutes! We are not usually interested in 'is there a difference?' so much as 'is there an important difference?'.

Remember this point:

Statistical significance has nothing whatsoever to do with practical significance.

Imagine for one moment that in the last problem μ_1 was actually 8·0005 and μ_0 was 8·0000. If we collected a large enough sample we could eventually shrink the 95% c.i. around μ_1 until it excluded μ_0 (e.g. for a sample of 100 million the 95% c.i.

would be approximately 8·0002–8·0008). We have, by sheer perseverance, demonstrated a 'statistically significant' difference between μ_1 and μ_0. Whether it was worth the effort is questionable: certainly a difference of 0·0005u/l would be of no practical significance if the variables were serum insulin concentrations in the populations of adult males and adult females!

The moral of this example is of fundamental importance— before embarking on an experiment of the sort described, ask yourself exactly how big a difference it is important for you to detect. Once that is decided upon you can proceed to determine the sample-size required to test the null hypothesis with a predetermined probability of detecting the difference if it in fact exists.

7.5. SAMPLE SIZE

The problem can be looked at like this. There are two possible ways of arriving at an incorrect conclusion on the basis of a hypothesis test.

First, we may obtain a 'statistically significant' result when the null hypothesis is in fact correct. This is a *type I* or α-error; a 'false positive' if you like!

Second, we may obtain a non-significant result when the null hypothesis is in fact incorrect. This is a *type II* or β-error; a 'false negative'.

The possible conclusions are summarized in *Table 12*.

Table 12

	H_0 true	H_0 false
Accept H_0	Correct decision	Type II error. probability = β
Reject H_0	Type I error. probability = α	Incorrect decision

To test the null hypothesis in a thoroughly scientific manner we should specify the risk we are prepared to take of both a type I and a type II error.

The *probability* of a type I error is the *significance level* of the test, α.

The *probability* of a type II error, β, given a specified probability for α (say 5%) *is determined by the size of the sample.* The quantity $1 - \beta$ is called the *power* of the test and in general we would like this to be as large as possible. Since power is directly related to β, it is apparent that power of the test (its sensitivity to differences) is directly related to the sample size n.

In order to determine the minimum sample size necessary for a particular test we must be able to specify:

$|\mu_1 - \mu_0|$, the absolute difference we want to detect if it exists;

   α, the significance level of the test. The probability we are prepared to accept of being wrong in saying a difference exists when it does not;

   β, the probability we are prepared to accept of failing to detect a difference when it in fact exists; and

   σ, the standard deviation of the test population distribution. An estimate S will suffice, based on a pilot study of at least 30 observations.

Calculate the Standard Normal deviate Q, were $Q = |\mu - \mu_0|/S$ Substitute this quantity into expression 7.3,

$$\text{minimum sample size, } n = (Z_{0.5-\alpha/2} + Z_{0.5-\beta})^2/Q^2. \qquad (7.3)$$

(from Natrella, 1960). The calculation is not as fearsome as it looks. Suppose that we set both α and β to 5%. In this case $Z_{0.5-\alpha/2}$ is the standard Normal deviate associated with the tabulated value of $0.5 - \alpha/2$, found in Appendix, *Table B*, e.g. $Z = (0.5 - 0.05/2) = 0.475$. Locate this value in the body of *Table B* and read off the corresponding standard unit, i.e. 1.96. The value for $Z_{0.5-\beta}$ is obtained in exactly the same way, i.e. 1.64.

Example 7.4

Using example 7.1 for illustration, we will suppose that we are only interested in differences of 1.0 or more between the test population mean and the theoretical mean μ_0, and that a pilot study provides us with $S = 1.58$.
Therefore:

$$Q = 1\cdot0/1\cdot58 = 0\cdot63,$$
$$\text{and } n = (1\cdot96 + 1\cdot64)^2/0\cdot63^2 = 32.$$

Conclusion:
In order to detect a difference of at least $1\cdot0$ between the test population mean μ_1 and the theoretical mean μ_0, we would require a sample of at least 32 observations, accepting in the process a probability of 5% for both type I and type II errors.

If we were comparing *two independent sample means*, as opposed to one sample mean and a known parameter, the calculation is very simply modified. We require good estimates of each population variance (using sample estimates from pilot studies) which we will call $S_A{}^2$ and $S_B{}^2$. The analysis assumes the underlying population parameters $\sigma_A{}^2$ and $\sigma_B{}^2$ to be equal. In practice the test can still be employed as a useful *approximation* by pooling the estimates as $\sqrt{(S_A{}^2 + S_B{}^2)}$. Q is calculated as follows:

$$Q = |\mu_A - \mu_B|/\sqrt{(S_A{}^2 + S_B{}^2)} \tag{7.4}$$

where $|\mu_A - \mu_B|$ is the minimum absolute difference between the two population means that we would like to detect, if it exists. Substitute Q into expression 7.3 and proceed as before, *multiplying the final result by two.*

7.6. COMPARING TWO SAMPLE MEANS (H_0: $\mu_1 = \mu_2$)
Given two sample means we may be interested in establishing whether or not the difference observed between them is compatible with identical underlying parameters ($\mu_1 = \mu_2$), or, more realistically, values of μ_1 and μ_2 that differ by less than some specified amount. This problem is complicated by the fact that we now have two sources of sampling variation. We could calculate 95% c.i. for each sample: if they clearly do not overlap our question is answered, i.e. we could reject H_0 out of hand. If they do overlap we have a statistical problem. Are we dealing with two samples with different sample $\bar{x}$ values but a common underlying population mean μ_0; or, two samples drawn from distinctly different populations μ_1 and μ_2? The situation is summarized in *Fig. 36.*

The classical approaches to testing H_0: $\mu_1 = \mu_2$ take quite a number of different forms depending upon the sample sizes involved, what we know of σ_1 and σ_2 or S_1 and S_2 and whether or not $\sigma_1 = \sigma_2$. Normal distributions are assumed throughout.

This is one occasion when a non-parametric significance test positively recommends itself for use. The *Fisher–Yates Normal Scores test* is one of the most powerful non-parametric tests described. It has nearly the same efficiency as the *t*-tests on Normally distributed data and is *more* efficient with non-Normal data (Kendall and Stuart, 1973).

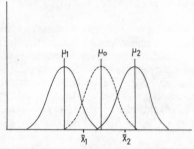

Fig. 36. Possible population structures underlying two sample means ($\bar{x}_1$ and $\bar{x}_2$).

It is no more complicated than a standard *t*-test and makes *no* assumptions about the sample data other than that samples should be independent of each other. The *t*-tests are simple enough to perform, once the appropriate form has been selected but their use demands some preliminary investigation of the data to ensure that it meets the test assumptions. It is one thing to say the *t*-tests are 'robust' to moderate departures from Normality, quite another to know just how far you can press your luck before the test misleads you.

An application of the Normal Scores test follows. The result of the test is given as an exact probability (α) which is generally preferable to a blind adherence to arbitrary 5% and 1% 'rejection' levels.

Example 7.5: Normal Scores (Fisher–Yates) test

Consider two samples, A and B of sizes $n_1 = 10$ and $n_2 = 15$ respectively, with a total number $n = 25$, i.e. $n_1 + n_2$

Our *null hypothesis* H_0 is that the two samples were drawn from populations having the same *mean* μ_0.

The *alternative hypothesis* H_1 is that the two samples were drawn from populations having *different* means μ_1 and μ_2

Data

Sample A: 4·0 3.3 2·2 3·2 0·8 1·7 0·6 1·1 3·1 1·4
Sample B: 2·0 4·8 2·6 2·1 2·6 1·6 4·4 2·5 4·4 2·7 4·3 1·8 4·5 3·6 2·2

Procedure

First, rank all of the values in ascending order of magnitude, writing under each value the letter A or B to indicate from which group the value originated.

TIE

0·6	0·8	1·1	1·4	1·6	1·7	1·8	2·0	2·1	2·2	2·2	2·5	2·6
A	A	A	A	B	A	B	B	B	B	A	B	B

2·6	2·7	3·1	3·2	3·3	3·6	4·0	4·3	4·4	4·4	4·5	4·8
B	B	A	A	A	B	A	B	B	B	B	B

The sequence of A's and B's is termed the *rank* sequence. Locate $n = 25$ in part A of the Normal Scores tables (Appendix, *Table G*) and write under each letter of the rank sequence the corresponding Normal Score with a negative sign; at the half-way point reverse the order of the Normal Scores and use a positive sign. The example should clarify this procedure:

A	A	A	A	B	A	B	B
−1·965	−1·524	−1·263	−1·067	−0·905	−0·764	−0·637	−0·519

B	B	A	B	B	B	B	A
−0·409	−0·303	−0·200	−0·099	0·00	+0·099	+0·200	+0·303

A	A	B	A	B	B	B	B	B
+0·409	+0·519	+0·637	+0·764	+0·905	+1·067	+1·263	+1·524	+1·965

The tied value is dealt with by averaging the two Normal Scores and using this for both A and B. Calculate the A-Score as the sum of the underlined A-scores.

(tie average)

$$\text{A-Score} = -1·965 -1·524 -1·263 -1·067 -0·764 -0·252$$
$$+0·303 +0·409 +0·519 +0·764 = -4·840.$$

Calculate the *variance* as $\dfrac{n_1 \cdot n_2}{n \cdot (n-1)} \cdot \Sigma S_i^2$.

The term ΣS_i^2 is obtained from part B of the Normal Scores tables. For this example $n = 25$ which has a tabulated value for ΣS_i^2 of 22·61046.

$$\text{Variance} = \left[\frac{10 \times 15}{25 \times 24}\right] \times 22 \cdot 61046 = 5 \cdot 6526.$$

Calculate the standardized Normal Scores Statistic
$Z = (\text{A-Score} - 0)/\sqrt{\text{Variance}}$:

$$Z = (-4 \cdot 840 - 0)/\sqrt{5 \cdot 6526} = -2 \cdot 04.$$

Locate the value Z in a table of the Normal probability integral (Appendix, *Table B*), i.e. look up 2·0 in the left-hand column and read across to 4. The tabulated value is 0·4793.

The *Test Probability*	=	(0·5 – tabulated integral) × 2
	=	(0·5 – 0·4793) × 2
	=	0·041.

Conclusion
Formally we reject H_0: $\mu_1 = \mu_2$ at a 4% significance level in favour of H_1. In plain English, the probability of observing sample means as different as those of samples A and B, *if* the null hypothesis were true, is only 4%. The evidence appears to support the alternative hypothesis, that the samples were in fact drawn from different populations. If we accept this conclusion we must also accept a 4·1% chance of being wrong in so doing.

7.7. PAIRED COMPARISONS
Experimental situations often arise in which samples are not independent of each other. We may have a randomly selected sample of five year old schoolchildren upon whom we measure serum immunoglobulin E levels immediately and again one year later. We would like to know if there is any significant difference between the two sets of results. The assumption of independence so essential to the previous means tests, has been lost. We have exactly the same children in both sample groups! A child who has a predisposition to low IgE levels will probably contribute a low result to both sets of results. The variation between children which is common to both sets of results tends to over-whelm the numerically smaller variation *between* results in the same children.

A second example might be the measurement of, for example, α-fetoprotein concentration in a set of amniotic fluids by two different assay methods. We would like to know if the assay methods give comparable results, or whether they differ in some consistent way. Once again the marked variation between the actual amniotic fluid concentrations tends to obscure the much smaller variation between the *estimated* concentrations of any individual specimen. Although this last example serves to illustrate the type of experimental situation in which independence is lost, it is in itself a good deal more complicated than it at first appears. Method comparison studies receive the exclusive attention of Chapter 10.

If we were to test $H_0: \mu_1 = \mu_2$ against $\mu_1 \neq \mu_2$ using the sample means, it is highly probable that we would fail to detect systematic differences between the paired values.

A more appropriate test would examine the differences between the paired values which *are* independent of each other. If these were quite random their expected mean would be zero. We test the null hypothesis $H_0: \mu_{1j} - \mu_{2j} = 0$ where j is each individual in the sample group.

The most appropriate analysis would be a two-way analysis of variance; but this requires a fairly sound statistical background. A popular analysis of the problem employs the *paired t-test*, and this is illustrated below on an artificially small sample.

Example 7.6
We have five subjects on each of whom we have plasma cortisol concentrations before and after a specific stress.

H_0: plasma cortisol levels are not affected by stress:

$\quad (H_0: \mu_{1j} - \mu_{2j} = 0)$

H_1: plasma cortisol levels are affected by stress:

$\quad (H_1: \mu_{1j} - \mu_{2j} \neq 0)$

Plasma Cortisol					
Subject	Pre-stress	Post-stress	difference, d	$d - \bar{d}$	$(d - \bar{d})^2$
1	400	440	40	7·4	54·76
2	560	590	30	−2·6	6·76
3	480	515	35	2·4	5·76
4	312	330	18	−14·6	213·16
5	700	740	40	7·4	54·76
$n = 5$			$\Sigma d = 163$	0·00	$\Sigma = 335 \cdot 20$

$\qquad\qquad\qquad\qquad\qquad\qquad\qquad\qquad \uparrow$
$\qquad\qquad\qquad\qquad\qquad \bar{d} = 32 \cdot 6 \quad$ Check on
$\qquad\qquad\qquad\qquad\qquad\qquad\qquad\quad$ arithmetic

$$S^2{}_D = \Sigma(d-\bar{d})^2/(n-1) = 335{\cdot}20/4 = 83{\cdot}80.$$

A 95% c.i. on the population difference Δ between the two groups is given by:

$$\begin{aligned}
95\% \text{ c.i. on } \Delta &= \bar{d} \pm t_{n-(10{\cdot}05)} \times \sqrt{(S_D{}^2/n)} \qquad (7.5)\\
&= 32{\cdot}6 \pm 2{\cdot}78 \times \sqrt{(83{\cdot}8/5)}\\
&= 21{\cdot}22\text{--}43{\cdot}98.
\end{aligned}$$

The 95% c.i. does not encompass zero, so we have some grounds for rejecting H_0 in favour of H_1, with a 5% probability of being wrong in so doing. It we required rather stronger evidence we could examine the 99% c.i. by substituting the tabulated value $t_{n-1(0{\cdot}01)}$ into expression 7.5:

$$\begin{aligned}
99\% \text{ c.i. on } \Delta &= \bar{d} \pm 4{\cdot}6 \times \sqrt{(83{\cdot}8/5)}\\
&= 13{\cdot}77\text{--}51{\cdot}43.
\end{aligned}$$

Since this interval still excludes zero, the evidence for rejecting H_0 appears to be quite convincing. It is unlikely (less than a 1:100 probability) that the observed differences between the two sample groups has arisen by chance (random sampling variation!) Note carefully the cautious conclusion, i.e. that there is a difference. *Not*, that the difference is due to stress. Without an adequate experimental design including a stress-free control group, the observed difference could just as easily be ascribed to circadian rhythm.

A test on the two sample means reveals *no* significant difference at the 5% probability level for α; (Normal Scores test) confirming the inadequacy of mean(s) tests when independence is lost.

Note: The paired t-test examines paired sample data for evidence of a constant difference. *If* the difference is dependent in some way upon the sample values, e.g. the difference between μ_{1j} and μ_{2j} is a percentage of μ_j, then a regression analysis (*see* Chapter 8) would be more appropriate than the paired t-test.

This is a good example of a situation in which several quite different statistical techniques could be brought to bear on a single problem, i.e. we could use a two way ANOVA, a paired t-test or a regression analysis, depending on the exact question being put to the paired sample data.

7.8. ONE-SIDED or TWO-SIDED

Sometimes we are not interested in the question 'is there a difference?' but rather 'is there an increase?'. We may have good theoretical or practical grounds for believing a particular difference between two parameters to be unlikely, e.g. if μ_1 is not equal to μ_2 it can only be lower.

Consider the paired t-test *example 7.6*. It is well established that stress induces cortisol synthesis and secretion. For the problem considered all we were really interested in was H_0: no change ($\mu_{2j} = \mu_{1j}$) and H_1: an *increase* ($\mu_{2j} > \mu_{1j}$).

By concentrating our examination of the experimental data for evidence of a specific alternative (an increase, as opposed to a change), whilst retaining a 5% significance level for the test, the corresponding probability of β (the type II error) is decreased. We have a *more powerful* test.

Practically, all that is required is to double the significance level we require, locate the corresponding t-value in *Table F* of Appendix 1 and set up the c.i. as before. If we want a 5% significance level with a *specific* alternative hypothesis, we set up a 90% c.i. and examine the side of the interval appropriate to H_1. For H_1: $\mu_{2j} > \mu_{1j}$ we are only interested in an increase in cortisol levels, a positive difference from zero, so we examine only the lower limit of the 90% c.i. (which has a 5% significance limit).

It is absolutely essential to define H_0 and H_1 *before* you collect the experimental results. This rather restricts the use of one-sided tests since it is not common for us to be absolutely certain that changes can occur in one direction only. We were presuming quite a lot for the cortisol experiment! Do not be tempted to specify a one-sided alternative *after* collecting the data (having presumably observed a specific trend up or down). The significance test assumes above all that the data are randomly sampled. As soon as you employ information from the experimental data to modify the analysis of that same information you are asking for real trouble. It's a little like predicting rain after you've got soaking wet!

7.9. MORE THAN TWO SAMPLES

Hypothesis tests on two samples can be readily extended to deal with more complicated problems involving three or more means. The process can be visualized as an extension of the ideas developed so far.

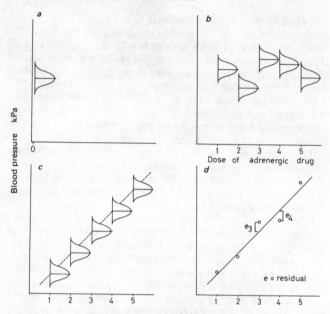

Fig. 37. Response patterns of blood pressure to increasing doses of an α-adrenergic drug.

Figure 37a exhibits the frequency distribution of blood pressures measured on a sample of individuals from some specified population. This might be the initial stage of the experiment, getting a 'feel' for the data we will be working with, its distributional properties, its mean and variability under sampling conditions.

We now take five random samples from this same population and administer increasing doses of a new α-adrenergic drug to each group, leaving the fifth group as an untreated control. The blood pressures in each group are recorded ten minutes after the introduction of the drug and the frequency distributions recorded in *Fig. 37b*. For samples we would expect some sampling variation in the observed group means. What we would like to know is whether the differences observed between the means are greater than can be reasonably accounted for by the sampling variation. The technique of analysis is the ANOVA (analysis of variance).

For the conclusions of the analysis to be valid we must take great care to exclude sources of variation other than the drug itself. If you felt so inclined you could argue (quite reasonably) that because group 2 were all given their doses of the drug by a particularly attractive nurse, the increased blood pressures observed ten minutes later have a perfectly simple explanation!

In order to isolate the 'treatment' effect the ANOVA technique has been integrated into a wide variety of mathematically based experimental designs. This is a truly vast area of statistical analysis with a large amount of specialized literature. The fundamental principles underlying the designs are: a) randomization; b) replication; c) blocking; d) covariate analysis.

Although the designs generally give rise to simple (if tedious) calculations, the process of selecting the most appropriate design for the problem at hand requires some skill and experience. Experiments are usually expensive, be it in time or money. If the culmination of a four year study involving hundreds, perhaps thousands of hospital patients, is the realization that the results are worthless because of an inadequate or inappropriate experimental design, you might appreciate the necessity for a careful analysis of the potential statistical problems *before* the experiment ever gets started. A very readable introduction to the whole area of experimental design is listed in the references (Cox, 1958).

Returning to our own experiment with the α-adrenergic drug, suppose that a significant difference between the sample group means has been established. The next question that might occur to the analyst is to ask whether or not the differences observed are related in any way to the dose of the drug given, i.e. is the statistically significant (and practically significant if we set the experiment up correctly) variation in the mean blood-pressures 'explained' by the experimentally controlled variation in drug dosage. The pattern of response in *Fig. 37c* suggests very strongly that there is a relation, and sets the scene for the next chapter, Regression Analysis.

REFERENCES

Cox D. R. (1958) *Planning of Experiments*. New York, Wiley.

Kendall M. G. and Stuart A. (1973) *The Advanced Theory of Statistics* Vol 2. London and High Wycombe, Griffin.

Natrella M. G. (1963) *Experimental Statistics N.B.S. Handbook 91*. Washington D.C., U.S. Govt. Printing Office.

8 Relationships

8.1. INTRODUCTION

Relationships between two sets of variables (x_i and y_i) can assume an infinite variety of forms under the general description $y = f(x)$. By far the commonest substitution for f is the straight-line function:

$$y = \alpha + \beta x$$

where α and β are the parameters of the straight-line relation, *Fig. 38*.

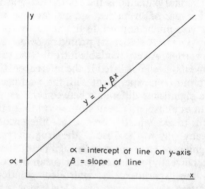

α = intercept of line on y-axis
β = slope of line

Fig. 38. Parameters of the straight-line relation.

The variable on the x-axis is sometimes called the 'independent' variable, whilst that on the y-axis is called the 'dependent' variable. This terminology is quite unrelated to the statistical use of the word 'independent'; it is a hand-me-down from graph theory and best avoided.

A second caution on terminology concerns the use of the word 'linear'. Straight-line relations are often described as linear relations, and as far as it goes this is quite correct. However, the

116

word linear can also be applied to the expression $y = \alpha + \beta_1 x + \beta_2 x^2$ which describes a quadratic curve, which is anything but a straight line! The quadratic expression is *linear in its parameters* α, β_1 and β_2, an essentially mathematical property. Textbooks often assume this technical use of the word linear to be known which can make life quite difficult for the uninitiated reader. If you want to say straight-line then just say that!

The analysis of non-linear relationships (in the mathematical sense) is quite an advanced topic. A good reason for modifying experimental conditions or results (by transformation) so that they fit straight-line models, is the desire to avoid the statistical and mathematical problems of a non-linear analysis.

Computers have opened up the field of non-linear analysis, mainly by taking charge of the extremely complicated and repetitive calculations involved, and these more complicated models have a natural appeal to the scientist who knows only too well that nature rarely works in a straight-line fashion. The theory however remains a serious obstacle to the non-mathematician.

The straight-line models, apart from being a good deal more straightforward to comprehend, possess the considerable virtue of having been in use for many years. The consequences of violating their assumptions are, for the most part, quite well known. Since experimental results rarely behave exactly as the textbooks would have them behave, it is useful to know what you can and cannot get away with in dealing with real-life data. Certainly, some statistical assumptions are less important than others, depending on the ultimate object of the analysis.

8.2. RELATIONSHIPS

Relationships between pairs of variables can be broadly categorized as follows:

1. Fundamentally *exact relations* which may or may not be obscured by observational or measurement errors in one, or both, of the variables involved. The underlying relation is mathematically exact, the product of a scientific law or theory. The only statistical interest stems from the uncertainty in the measurements made on that law. For example, Beer's law defines an exact linear relation between the light absorbtion of a chromogen in solution and the concentration of the chromogen. Measurements of the absorbtion may range from crudely

approximate to highly precise, depending on the instrument used. If the solutions are artificially prepared, the stated concentrations will certainly be subject to some error, although one would hope that this was negligible (don't be too quick to assume that it is—what is the imprecision of *your* 'precision' balance?).

2. *Law-like relations* in which a clear relationship appears to underlie the data but which cannot be completely specified mathematically because of an *inherent* random element in one or both of the variables involved. This might itself be further obscured by measurement errors. For example, there is a definite relationship between the haemoglobin concentration of blood and altitude. People who live up in the mountains have higher haemoglobin concentrations, better to utilize the reduced amount of available oxygen. The manner in which this relationship arises is biologically complicated and unlikely to yield to exact specification in mathematical terms. In addition, individuals vary a great deal with respect to their haemoglobin concentrations, lending a distinct statistical element to what is essentially a real, physical relationship. Finally, haemoglobin concentrations in blood cannot be measured without appreciable error.

3. Essentially statistical relationships in which a law-like process is unlikely to be discerned, either because it does not exist, or because it is embedded in, and a part of, a complicated network of interacting random variables, e.g., intelligence and income. These relationships are better described as *associations* and may be useful for the purpose of prediction, as a justification for further more detailed study or as the starting point for a variety of multivariate analyses aimed at identifying patterns or structure in complex situations.

The groupings 1, 2 and 3 are themselves an attempt to impose structure upon what is in reality a continuous spectrum of variation in relationships from the mathematically exact to the statistically nebulous. The way we approach any particular problem is determined to quite a large extent by the ultimate objective of our analysis. For this reason it is worthwhile devoting a substantial proportion of the time allocated to an experimental programme to clarifying its objectives and identifying the nature of the experimental variables involved. The *statistical model* assumed for the situation under study is determined by these factors: the more time and trouble that is taken to model the situation correctly, the greater the likelihood of obtaining an unambiguous conclusion to the study, using data appropriate to the model.

Modifications to the experimental protocol, some well-planned randomizations, and a little strategic replication, may be all that is required to permit the use of a simple model for which a straightforward and elegant analysis is available.

Model first, data next, statistical analysis last.

8.3 MODELLING STRAIGHT-LINE RELATIONSHIPS

1. The simplest straight-line model is the exact linear functional relation:

$$y = \alpha + \beta x.$$

This relationship is characteristic of a number of physical laws: Boyle's law, Hooke's law, Beer's law. The last will be familiar to most laboratory personnel, describing as it does the relationship between the light absorbtion (A) of a solution and the concentration (C) of the absorbing chromogen in that solution, in the form $A = \Delta CL$, illustrated in *Fig. 39a*.

Δ is the molar extinction coefficient and L is the length of the absorbing light path. If L is fixed in length (say 1 cm), the equation reduces to:

$$A = \Delta \cdot C$$

corresponding to $y = \alpha + \beta \cdot x$, where $\alpha = 0$.

If we could establish both the concentration and the absorbance for a set of absorbing solutions without any appreciable error, the pairs of measurements x_i and y_i would fall exactly on a straight line. We could fit a straight line with a ruler and determine its slope β (equivalent to Δ) exactly, by trivial arithmetic.

2. A more realistic situation is one in which we have a set of solutions whose concentrations are known exactly, since they were prepared under controlled conditions in the laboratory, i.e. 'standard' solutions or 'calibrators'. However, the instrument used to record the absorbance of these calibrators is imprecise, subject to small but detectable fluctuations. Instead of recording the true absorbance associated with any particular calibrator, we can observe only one of a range of values in the vicinity of the true value. The fluctuations are generally symmetrical about the true absorbance and theoretical considerations (the central limit theorem) suggest that their distribution may well be approximately Normal.

We have, in effect, an exact linear functional relation under-lying the observed values, between the means $\bar{y}_i$ (the true absor-bances), and the known calibrator concentrations x_i. The situa-tion is summarized in expression 8.1 and *Fig. 39a*.

$$\bar{y}_i = \alpha + \beta x_i. \tag{8.1}$$

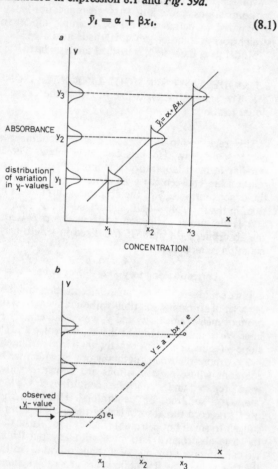

Fig. 39. The simple linear regression model. *Note:* α = zero here.

The problem is that we are rarely in a position to take several hundred measurements (y_i) for each concentration (x_i), thereby establishing the values of α and β for the *exact* relation of expression 8.1.

In reality we may have only *one* measurement y_i for each x_i, the situation represented in *Fig. 39b*.

The y_i measurements are composed of two parts, the underlying true absorbance $\bar{y}_i$ (which is exactly related to x_i), and a fluctuating part ε_i (the measurement error) attributable to analytical imprecision. The fluctuating part ε_i is described in general terms as the disturbance term and is given by:

$$\varepsilon_i = y_i - \bar{y}_i.$$

The underlying exact relation of expression 8.1 is actually observed as follows:

$$y_i = \alpha + \beta x_i + \varepsilon_i. \tag{8.2}$$

So long as the individual y_i measurements are symmetrically distributed about their respective means $\bar{y}_i$, the parameters α and β of expressions 8.1 and 8.2 remain identical.

The practical problem that confronts us is this. The experimental data points $x_i y_i$ no longer fall in an exact straight-line when plotted on a graph. The larger the disturbance terms ε_i (the measurement errors in this case) the greater the scatter of the data points about the underlying relation of 8.1, until it becomes very much a matter of opinion as to how to draw the 'best' straight-line through the points. The best straight-line is one whose observed y-intercept (denoted by a) and slope (denoted by b) are as close as possible to the underlying parameters α and β. We require a means of calculating consistent, unbiased and efficient estimates (*see* section 7.2) of the parameters α and β.

The classical solution is to fit a straight-line in such a way that the squared distances of the data points ($x_i y_i$) from the fitted line (parallel to the y-axis) are at a minimum. This is called the line of least-squares and is an essentially arithmetical technique. If we are prepared to make a number of assumptions about the distributional properties of the disturbance terms ε_i, the technique of least-squares becomes transformed into a principle of statistical estimation for α and β, its estimates a and b having all of the properties we require.

Using the least-squares principle on sample (experimental) data, we calculate a sample line of the form:

$$Y_i = a + b \cdot x_i + e_i, \qquad (8.3)$$

where e_i is the distance between the observed y_i values and the fitted least-squares line (8.3). The quantity e_i is referred to as a *residual* (the 'residual' variation about the fitted line), and can be calculated directly from the original experimental data as the difference between the *experimental* y_i values and the *predicted* Y_i values obtained by substitution of the calibrator concentrations x_i in equation (8.3)

$$e_i = y_i - Y_i. \qquad (8.4)$$

The standard deviation of the residuals S_e can be calculated (*see* section 8.6) and is an estimate of the standard deviation of the disturbance term ε_i. The residual is an extremely important quantity in evaluating how well the model of expression 8.3 describes the experimental reality (... model's are by definition false!) Confidence intervals for α, β and $\bar{y}_i$ can be constructed from the sample statistics a, b and S_e (*see* section 8.6).

> *To summarize:*
>   *We postulate:* $\bar{y}_i = \alpha + \beta x_i$
>   *We work with:* $y_i = \alpha + \beta x_i + \varepsilon_i$
>
> (where $\varepsilon_i = y_i - \bar{y}_i$, a disturbance term attributable to measurement error, biological variation or both:)
>
>   *Which we estimate as:* $Y_i = a + b x_i + e_i$
>
> (where $e_i = y_i - Y_i$, the residual variation about the least-squares line).

Note: It is entirely possible that in a different experimental situation to the one described, the y_i variable is observed without any measurement error at all to speak of, but that it exhibits an inherent random fluctuation. For example, in *Fig. 39* the x-variable could represent fixed doses for an α-adrenergic drug (accurately known) whilst the y-variable represents the blood pressures recorded in a suitably randomized group of recipients of the drug.

The higher the dose of the drug, the higher the blood pressure recorded. We postulate an exact relation between mean blood pressure and drug dose but we are obliged to work with the somewhat inexact relation between the recorded blood pressure, in a limited sample of test subjects, and the drug dose.

The disturbance term ε_i in this situation tells us that different individuals receiving the same dose of drug exhibit somewhat different elevations in their blood pressures. This hardly constitutes an 'error'. It is simply the natural random, or biological, variation between individuals, despite all attempts made to 'standardize' them in originally defining the population of interest. The mean values y_i are no longer 'true' values, simply the average response to the drug in the population under study.

Just to complicate the issue we may only be able to record the blood pressures approximately for one reason or another. The disturbance term ε_i will now represent the combined effects of biological variation and measurement error!

3. More complicated models arise when both the x and y variables are subject to observation or measurement error.

If the underlying model is an exact functional relation (*see* 8.3, 1., above) such as that of Beer's law, but both absorbance and concentration are recorded with random errors of measurement, the model obtained is a *functional errors-in-variables model*. If one (or both) of the variables has an inherent random element, e.g. the relationship between the dose of a drug and blood pressure, and both are recorded approximately (they both have random measurement errors), the model obtained is a *structural errors-in-variables model*.

These are rather complicated models but they have considerable relevance to the medical laboratory, where measurement error is a daily fact of life. Consideration of the errors-in-variables models will be deferred to the chapter on method comparison studies (Chapter 10).

4. For the simple linear regression model we selected specific values of one variable x (no random elements at all) and recorded the values of a corresponding variable y (random, either intrinsically or as a consequence of errors of observation). This model is most appropriate to a good deal of experimental research where the analyst can control one variable (x) artificially and record the resulting response of the uncontrolled variable (y).

In many situations such control is not practical (or even possible!) and the research may then take the form of a sampling study. Subjects are selected at random from a defined population and the values of two random variables x and y recorded for each subject, e.g. height and weight. Both are completely random and are described by a joint or bivariate probability distribution (*see Figs. 23* and *24*). If both random variables involved are Normally distributed, the joint distribution is referred to as *bivariate Normal.* The relationship we are looking at is fundamentally different from those previously considered. Being uncontrolled, it is essentially statistical in nature. All we are usually interested in is the evidence of an empirical association between the two variables. We might use such evidence for description, prediction or as the basis for more carefully controlled studies on the variables.

It is very risky inferring a causal basis for the observed associations of sampling studies, as the controversy over smoking and cancer illustrates. The evidence of sampling studies is always open to the criticism that the two groups studied, say smokers and non-smokers, differ in some less obvious respect that *actually* explains the differing incidence of bronchial carcinomas, e.g. diet, genetic constitution, anxiety (about the cost of smoking) or anything else you may care to think of.

All of the non-cigarette variables between the smoking and non-smoking groups could be controlled in a well-organized randomized experimental design using a group of young children. Half of the group could be assigned as non-smoking controls, the other half split into sub-groups of increasing cigarette consumption. By maintaining the experimental conditions for the whole group for forty years the arguments could be resolved quite effectively. Either the smoking group exhibits a significantly higher incidence of bronchial carcinoma than the identically treated controls, or it does not! The only difference between the two groups is the cigarette variable.

Buried in the experimental design we had a simple regression model, x (fixed) = number of cigarettes smoked per day and y (variable) = incidence of bronchial carcinoma. If a statistically significant relationship were to be demonstrated it would be powerful evidence for a causal relation. There are many situations in which ethics, economics or simple ignorance oblige us to make the best we can of sampling research. It is as well to remember the fragile nature of the evidence they provide.

The hidden variable underlying many observed associations is time. The declining whale population of the world's oceans is strongly associated (on a graph) with the consumption of tranquillizers. One is going down whilst the other is going up. It would be nice to postulate that all those anxious people were in fact worried about the fate of our Cetacean friends, but it seems, on reflection, to be unlikely! The 'third' variable to which the other two are closely related is time, whose passing is witness to many otherwise unrelated changes. The 'third' variable can often be very well concealed, so tread carefully in dealing with sampling associations.

The bivariate Normal distribution underlies the *bivariate regression model*, in which both x and y are random variables, each Normally distributed.

We will consider in the following sections the analysis of two models: the simple linear regression model; and the bivariate regression model. Much of the arithmetic of analysis is common to both models, resulting in considerable confusion between the two. The interpretation of the results for one model may lead to quite nonsensical conclusions when applied to another. The word regression is an historical curiosity that nowadays covers a multiplicity of models. Never use it without qualification.

8.4. SIMPLE LINEAR REGRESSION MODEL
There are a number of different reasons why the analyst might require estimates of the parameters α and β.

1. The sample statistics a and b provide a convenient statistical shorthand for summarizing two sets of related variables, in much the same way as the sample mean $\bar{x}$ and standard deviation S were used to summarize the single set of 300 values in *Table 1*.

2. If the underlying relationship is functional, the product of a physical or biochemical process, the parameters α and β may be interpretable as physical or biochemical constants. The analyst would like estimates of these constants in which he can have a specified degree of confidence.

3. The analyst may not be certain that a relationship exists at all. He would like to test the null hypothesis H_0: no relationship, against the alternative H_1: a straight-line relationship. This is equivalent to testing H_0: $\beta = 0$ against H_1: $\beta \neq 0$.

4. The analyst may wish to predict the mean response $\bar{y}$ for a given value of x_i, preferably with a confidence interval.

5. The analyst may require some indication of the range of predicted y_i values he is likely to observe in association with a particular x_i value. The interval required is for the predicted y_i values, *not* the underlying mean $\bar{y}_i$: it is sometimes described as a *tolerance interval* or a prediction interval.

6. In the clinical laboratory the simple linear regression model may be used to describe calibration lines for quantitative clinical assays. Having obtained an estimate of the calibration line, the analyst will want to use it to calculate the concentrations x_t (with appropriate confidence intervals) of patient's test samples, given absorbance readings y_t from those processed samples. This requires some rearrangement of the regression equation 8.3 and leads to a number of quite characteristic problems. This last situation is commonly referred to as the 'calibration problem'.

8.5. CHECKING THE MODEL ASSUMPTIONS

We have a non-random variable x (fixed by the experimenter) and a random variable y, the mean values of which ($\bar{y}_t$) are exactly related to x_t.

The assumptions we make for the simple linear regression model follow (see 1–6 below).

> (1). We assume that a straight-line relationship does in fact exist between the means $\bar{y}_t$ and the variable x_t.

Never forget to plot your experimental data points on a graph. The appearance of the graph conveys a lot of useful information, quite apart from preventing the description of obvious curves by straight-lines. If a computer is employed to perform the regression analyses, ensure that it provides you with a graphical output. The computer will fit a straight line to anything it is instructed to. It assumes you know what you are doing!

In some situations we may claim good theoretical grounds for believing the underlying relationship to be a straight-line, as in the case of Beer's law, discussed in section 8.3. In practice however, deviations from Beer's law are not uncommon so it pays to be critical.

Any really obvious departures from a straight-line will be picked up on the graph. Less obvious departures will require a little more thought. Depending on the ultimate objectives of your experiment you *may* be quite happy to accept the evidence of your own eyes from *Fig. 40a*. You get the level of approximation you ask for: if rough and ready is all you want, rough and ready is all you'll get!

Tests of the straight-line assumption are available and should be employed if the object of the analysis is anything more than a simple summary description of the data, e.g. estimation/

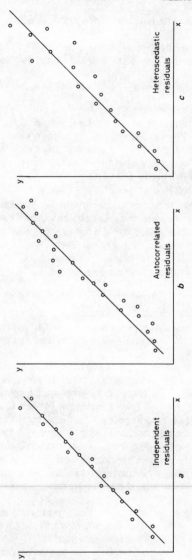

Fig. 40. Patterns of residual variation.

prediction. There are two main approaches to testing the straight-line assumption:

(i). If measurements/observations are made for ten or more x-values, we could try fitting a quadratic curve to the sample data:

$$Y_i = a + b_1x_i + b_2x_i{}^2 + e_i \qquad (8.5)$$

If the residual variation $(S_e{}^2)$ of the data points about the fitted curve were significantly smaller than the residual variation about a straight-line $Y_i = a + bx_i + e_i$, we might reasonably conclude that the curve of expression 8.5 was a more satisfactory model for approximating the experimental data. The risks of pursuing this approach with too few data points are discussed in the curvature section 9.9.

(ii). With less than ten points it will be necessary to obtain repeated measurements of y_i at each x_i value. The straight-line assumption is then tested using a modified ANOVA (see section 7.9). Both approaches are discussed with worked examples in Armitage (1974). If curvature is demonstrated, the techniques for dealing with it are discussed in section 9.9.

---

(2). We assume the disturbance terms ε_i to be Normally distributed.

The Normality assumption is equivalent to saying that the y_i values should be Normally distributed about their respective mean values $\bar{y}_i$, as shown in *Fig. 39a*.

The assumption is not essential for the simple fitting of a straight-line to the experimental data. If however the sample intercept a and slope b are to be employed for estimation (see section 7.1) of α and β (point or interval), then the assumption of Normality becomes important, particularly if the sample size is small. In common with the sample mean $\bar{x}$, the statistics a and b have sampling distributions that tend to Normality as the sample size increases, even when the original disturbance terms ε_i are not themselves Normally distributed. As a result, for large samples of experimental data, the Normality assumption is not critical.

If it is intended that the simple linear regression model be used for prediction of $\bar{y}_i$ or Y_i, with appropriate confidence intervals, the Normality assumption is quite critical.

The calculated residuals e_i from the original experimental data can be tested directly for Normality using the methods of section

4.5, assuming that enough values are available. Alternatively, repeated measurements of y should be taken at several different x_i values and tested directly for Normality.

> (3). We assume the standard deviation of the disturbance terms S_e to be constant for any given value of y_i, i.e. homoscedastic (see Fig. 28).

A graph of the experimental data is a valuable guide to the adequacy of this assumption. If the experimental data appears to have a reasonably uniform scatter throughout the measurement range, as in Fig. 40a, there is little cause for concern. In the graph Fig. 40c the scatter of the data points is clearly changing with the magnitude of y, i.e. it is heteroscedastic (see Fig. 29) and we have something of a problem.

The assumption of homoscedasticity is not essential for the calculation of the intercept a and slope b, nor for their use in point estimation of α and β, i.e. the estimates remain consistent and unbiased. They are however less efficient and if the analysis is important or if the construction of confidence and prediction intervals is planned, steps should be taken to test the homoscedasticity assumption.

Estimates of the residual variance S_e^2 are required at several points throughout the measurement range. These can be obtained from repeated measurements of the y-variable at fixed values of the x-variable. For three or more such variance estimates Bartlett's test for homogeneity of variance can be used. A worked example is given in Snedecor and Cochran (1974). It should be noted that this relatively simple test is itself critically dependent upon the assumption of Normality.

If a marked non-constant residual variation is established, two main courses of action are available:

(i). A *transformation* of the experimental data can be employed to stabilize the residual variance, i.e. render it homoscedastic. By and large this approach calls for some skill, particularly when it comes to back-transforming the estimated intercept and slope into the original measurement scale. Recall the problems associated with back-transforming a logarithmic mean in section 2.3. The effects of variance-stabilizing transformations on the Normality assumption also need to be carefully considered. You may be exchanging one problem for several larger ones! Some very practical advice is available in a paper by Healy (1968).

(ii). A *weighted* least-squares regression analysis can be employed that specifically accommodates an heteroscedastic disturbance term. This analysis requires estimates of the residual variance S_e^2 throughout the measurement range. In practice this demands a minimum of 10 replicate y measurements at every data point x_i if the S_e^2 estimates are to be of any value.

In the analysis itself, those y-values associated with a high degree of uncertainty (or imprecision: large variance) are given less importance in the calculation of the slope b than those y-values with a low degree of uncertainty (small variance). This principle underlies the original formulation of the least-squares principle, the simple least-squares regression model being a restricted version in which all of the residual variances are assumed to have a uniform 'weight' of 1. The subject is treated in thoroughly readable detail by Mandel (1964).

---

(4). We assume the disturbance term ε_i to be entirely due to random variation (or measurement error) in the y-variable. The x-variable is assumed to be known with complete certainty.

The consequences of a failure in this assumption are discussed in the context of a specific laboratory problem in chapter 10. In brief, the introduction of a disturbance term (or measurement error) into our x-variable means that the simple linear regression model is no longer a satisfactory representation of the experimental situation, and the calculated least-squares slope b will tend to underestimate the underlying slope β, i.e. the least-squares estimator of β is no longer unbiased.

A quite specific exception to the assumption has been identified by Berkson (1950). This is a situation in which the experimenter controls the x-variable by setting an instrument to predetermined values, recording the response of interest (y_i) at those values. The value of the x-variable recorded by the experimenter on his work-sheet will be the pre-determined value, since he will have set the instrument (balance, voltmeter, burette, etc.) to read exactly that value. The instrument may be imprecise but the reading recorded on the worksheet is not! If you suspect some sleight-of-hand in this statement, consider several repetitions of an experiment in which the experimenter sets an instrument to read 10, 20 and 30 volts respectively, at each of which levels a response y_i is measured. In every repetition of this experiment the recorded x-values are 10, 20 and 30 volts. There is no error at all in the *recorded* voltages. The subtlety involved is that we never recorded the actual voltage of the machine at all (which is subject to measurement error or imprecision), only the *intended* voltages required for the experiment, which do not vary at all. Under these conditions, the simple linear regression model is quite adequate since the x-variable, the intended values, are known with complete certainty. The price paid for using the Berkson model is that we sacrifice any insight we may have gained into the imprecision of the instrument used to set the x-values.

---

(5). The disturbance terms ε_t and assumed to be statistically independent, i.e. completely random.

Once again a graph of the experimental data is a valuable guide to the adequacy of the assumption. The residual variation of the data points about the fitted least-squares regression line in *Fig. 40a* appears to be quite random, whilst in *Fig. 40b* there is a distinct pattern to the scatter suggestive of autocorrelation, a primary departure from the independence assumption. This is most commonly associated with experiments in which the x-variable is time. However, in *Fig. 40b* the residual autocorrelation appears to be so regular that it may simply be an artefact induced by fitting a straight-line to data that would have been more satisfactorily described by a curve.

Testing residuals for randomness necessitates the initial calculation of the least-squares regression equation (described in section 8.6) so that the residuals e_t can be calculated for the experimental data.

Example 8.1

Experimental data:	x_t	y_t
	1	12·9
	2	15·1
	3	15·8
	4	17·7
	5	19·9

Least-squares estimates of $a = 11\cdot3$ and $b = 1\cdot66$, so that:

$$Y_t = 11\cdot3 + 1\cdot66x_t$$

If we substitute the experimental x_t values into this equation we can calculate the predicted Y_t values and in turn the residuals $e_t = y_t - Y_t$.

	Observed	Predicted	Residual
x_i	y_i	Y_i	e_i
1	12·9	12·96	−0·06
2	15·1	14·62	+0·48
3	15·8	16·28	−0·48
4	17·7	17·94	−0·24
5	19·9	19·60	+0·30
		Mean	= 0·00

Note: The residual standard deviation S_e can be calculated directly on the tabulated e_i values above using the standard deviation formula of expression 2·4, with $n - 2$ as a divisor instead of $n - 1$. Since the residual mean $\bar{e} = 0$, expression 2·4 can be simplified to:

$$S_e = \sqrt{[\Sigma e_i{}^2/(n - 2)]} = 0·4517.$$

The use of $n - 2$ as a divisor is not entirely straightforward to explain, but it can be pictured as follows. If we had only 2 data points, a best-fitting straight line would of necessity have to pass exactly through both points. There would be no 'information' available as to the adequacy of the straight-line model as an approximation of the reality underlying this rather inadequate sample of data, i.e. we have no residuals to assess the 'goodness-of-fit' of the model to the data. If 3 data points were available we would have one piece of 'information' available, i.e. $(n - 2)$, as to the goodness-of-fit. The argument extends to four or more data points. In general sample data contains a finite amount of information about the structure of the population from which it was drawn. Every time a population parameter is estimated from the sample data, we consume some of this information: in technical terms we lose 'a degree of freedom' for every parameter estimated from the sample data. To calculate the sample standard deviation S of expression 2·4, we had first to estimate the population mean μ using the sample mean $\bar{x}$, hence the loss of one degree of freedom $(n - 1)$. To calculate the linear regression residual S_e we had first to estimate two parameters α and β from the sample data, hence the loss of two degrees of freedom $(n - 2)$.

The residual standard deviation S_e can be calculated a great deal more quickly as is demonstrated in the worked regression example 8.2 of section 8.6.

The Durbin–Watson statistic d for autocorrelation examines the residuals e_t for evidence of non-randomness.

Durbin–Watson statistic $d = \Sigma(e_t - e_{t+1})^2/\Sigma e_t^2$

For the example problem we have:

$$d = \{(-0{\cdot}06 - 0{\cdot}48)^2 + [0{\cdot}48 - (-0{\cdot}48)]^2 + [-0{\cdot}48$$
$$- (-0{\cdot}24)]^2 + (-0{\cdot}24 - 0{\cdot}3)^2\}/\{(-0{\cdot}06)^2 + (0{\cdot}48)^2 +$$
$$(-0{\cdot}48)^2 + (-0{\cdot}24)^2 + (0{\cdot}3)^2\}$$
$$= 1{\cdot}5624/0{\cdot}612 = 2{\cdot}5529.$$

Note: If the test value is below 2 the calculation is complete. If the test value is in excess of 2, as above, subtract it from 4 to obtain the test statistic d, i.e. $4 - 2{\cdot}5529 = 1{\cdot}4471$.

In general, the closer the value d is to 2, the less cause we have to suspect a non-random residual variation. For samples of 15 or more observations, tables of critical values for the test statistic d are available (Neave, 1978). By way of illustration an abbreviated table of the 5% critical values follows (*Table 13*)—here $_L$ is for lower, u for upper value.

Table 13.

n	d_L	d_u
15	1·077	1·361
25	1·288	1·454
50	1·503	1·585
100	1·654	1·694

If the test statistic d is less than the tabulated value d_L for sample size n, we have some evidence for the existence of auto correlated residuals.

If the test statistic d falls between the values d_L and d_u the result is equivocal.

If the test statistic d is greater than the tabulated value d_u, we have no good evidence for the existence of autocorrelated residuals.

Even though our test sample consists of only five observations ($n = 5$), it is apparent that the calculated value of $d = 1{\cdot}4471$ is well above the critical value d_u for $n = 15$, suggesting that we have little cause to suspect non-randomness.

For small sample groups (less than 15), a rough and ready evaluation of the test statistic d can be obtained by referring the quantity $1 - (d/2)$ to tables of critical values of the correlation coefficient (Appendix, *Table E*). For example,

$$1 - (1{\cdot}4471/2) = 0{\cdot}2761.$$

From *Table E*, the critical value tabulated for $n = 5(p0{\cdot}05)$ is $0{\cdot}878$.

Since our modified test statistic $0{\cdot}2761$ is well below the critical value of $0{\cdot}878$, we confirm our previous conclusion that there is no evidence for non-randomness. Do bear in mind that this last device is a rough guide only for small samples.

(6). We assume there are no outliers in the sample data.

Outliers are data points which appear to differ markedly from the main body of the data. In *Fig. 42*, an outlier has been inserted on the graph purely for illustration. Outliers, or 'wild-points' are a contentious subject. *No* data should ever be excluded from the statistical analysis without sound technical justification, e.g. bacterial contamination of a test serum. If it looks unsightly on your graph, ask yourself how it got there, not how can you get rid of it! It is telling you something about the experimental set-up and your conclusions should acknowledge its occurrence It may be the only really interesting thing that happened in the entire study! There are no statistical grounds for excluding outliers.

Residual plots

A useful graphical device for checking the model assumptions is the residual plot, which can be recommended for samples of ten or more observations.

Divide each of the calculated residuals by the overall residual standard deviation S_e. Since the residual mean is zero this step is identical to the Standard Normal variable transformation of expression 4.2,

$$\text{Standardized residual } E_i = e_i/S_e \tag{8.6}$$

The standardized residuals (zero mean and unit standard deviation) are plotted against their corresponding x_i variables on a simple x–y graph with E_i on the y-axis. In general the standardized residuals should be randomly scattered about zero on the y-axis with the majority falling in the range -2 to $+2$ (*Fig. 41a, b, c*).

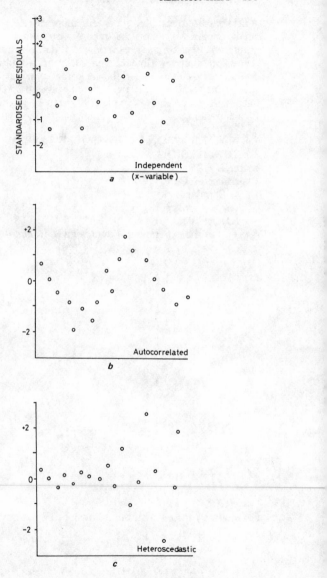

Fig. 41. Standardized residual plots corresponding to the patterns in *Fig. 40*.

Standardized residual plots are more effective in revealing small departures from the model assumptions than simple graphs of the original experimental data. Computer based regression analyses (linear, non-linear and multivariate) are considerably enhanced by the inclusion of a residual plotting subroutine, in addition to the absolutely essential basic graphical output. A paper by Anscombe (1973) can be recommended for further reading.

8.6. CALCULATIONS FOR SIMPLE LINEAR REGRESSION MODEL

Example 8.2
Experimental Data

Standard

x (Concentration mg/l) =	1	2	3	4	5
y (Optical density) =	0·18	0·43	0·55	0·82	0·96

A graph of the experimental data is given in *Fig. 42.*

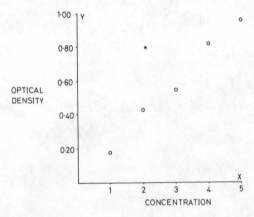

Fig. 42. Example 8.2.

Calculations

Familiarize yourself with the following summations:

$$\Sigma x = x_1 + x_2 + \ldots + x_n, \text{ where } n = \text{sample size}$$
$$\Sigma x^2 = x_1^2 + x_2^2 + \ldots + x_n^2$$
$$\Sigma xy = (x_1 \cdot y_1) + (x_2 \cdot y_2) + \ldots + (x_n \cdot y_n)$$

For the experimental data of example 8.2:

$$n = 5 \qquad x = \text{concentration}$$
$$\Sigma x = 15 \cdot 000 \qquad y = \text{optical density}$$
$$\Sigma x^2 = 55.000$$
$$\Sigma y = 2 \cdot 940$$
$$\Sigma y^2 = 2 \cdot 114$$
$$\Sigma xy = 10 \cdot 770$$
$$\bar{x} = 3 \cdot 000$$
$$\bar{y} = 0 \cdot 588$$

$$SS_x = 10 \cdot 000 \qquad SS_x = \Sigma x^2 - (\Sigma x)^2/n$$
$$SS_y = 0 \cdot 385 \qquad SS_y = \Sigma y^2 - (\Sigma y)^2/n$$
$$SS_{xy} = 1 \cdot 950 \qquad SS_{xy} = \Sigma xy - (\Sigma x \cdot \Sigma y)/n$$
$$S_x^2 = 2 \cdot 500 \qquad S_x^2 = SS_x/(n-1)$$
$$S_y^2 = 0 \cdot 096 \qquad S_y^2 = SS_y/(n-1)$$
$$S_x = 1 \cdot 581$$
$$S_y = 0 \cdot 310$$

We now have the basic tools required to answer each of the experimental questions outlined in section 8.4 (1 – 6).

Answering *8.4, 1*.

Sample slope $b = SS_{xy}/SS_x = 0 \cdot 195$; $\qquad$ (8.7)

Sample y-int. $a = \bar{y} - b \cdot \bar{x} = 0 \cdot 003$; $\qquad$ (8.8)

Sample residual
variance $S_e^2 = (SS_y - [(SS_{xy})^2/SS_x])/(n-2)$ $\qquad$ (8.9)
$= 0 \cdot 0016$;

Summary of
sample data: $Y = 0 \cdot 003 + 0 \cdot 195x$.

Answering *8.4, 2* and *8.4, 3*.

95 % c.i. on $\beta = b \pm [t_{n-2} \cdot \text{Standard error of } b]$
$= b \pm [t_{n-2} \cdot \sqrt{(S_e^2/SS_x)}]$ $\qquad$ (8.10)

Locate the required value of t in the *table F* (Appendix) by reading down the left-hand column to $n - 2$ (in this case $= 3$) and across to the 0·05 probability level. The tabulated value of t is 3·182. So, substituting,

95 % c.i. on $\beta = 0 \cdot 195 \pm [3 \cdot 182 \cdot \sqrt{(0 \cdot 0016/10)}]$
$= 0 \cdot 155 - 0 \cdot 235$.

There is a 95% probability that this interval encompasses the value of the population parameter β. Since the interval excludes zero there is, correspondingly, a less than 5% probability that $\beta = 0$. We have reasonable evidence for rejecting H_0: $\beta = 0$ in favour of H_1: $\beta \neq 0$, i.e. there appears to be a real relationship between x and y, the question of objective 8.4, 3.

95% c.i. on $\alpha = a \pm [t_{n-2} \cdot$ standard error of $a]$

$$= a \pm \left[t_{n-2} \cdot \sqrt{\left\{ S_e{}^2 \cdot \left(\frac{1}{n} + \frac{\bar{x}^2}{SS_x} \right) \right\}} \right] \quad (8.11)$$

$$= 0 \cdot 003 \pm \left[3 \cdot 182 \cdot \sqrt{\left\{ 0 \cdot 0016 \cdot \left(\frac{1}{5} + \frac{3 \cdot 00^2}{10} \right) \right\}} \right]$$

$$= -0 \cdot 130 - 0 \cdot 136.$$

The 95% c.i. on α encompasses zero, suggesting that the population parameter is quite compatible with a value of zero.

The objectives of 8.4, 2., the estimation of α and β, are now fulfilled. We have:

$$\text{point estimates } a = 0 \cdot 003,$$
$$b = 0 \cdot 198;$$

and interval estimates on $\alpha = -0 \cdot 130 - 0 \cdot 136$,

$$\text{and on } \beta = 0 \cdot 155 - 0 \cdot 235.$$

The objective of 8.4, 3. is satisfied from the interpretation of the 95% c.i. on β, i.e. β is significantly different from zero.

All that remain are the prediction intervals on $\bar{y}_t$ and Y_t.

Answering 8.4, 4.

A 95% c.i. on $\bar{y}_t$ for a given value of x:

say $x_t = 2 \cdot 5$. The estimated value of $Y_t = 0 \cdot 003 + (0 \cdot 195 \cdot 2 \cdot 5)$
$$= 0 \cdot 491.$$

95% c.i. on $\bar{y}_t = Y_t \pm t_{n-2} \sqrt{\left[S_e{}^2 \cdot \left(\frac{1}{n} + \frac{(x_t - \bar{x})^2}{SS_x} \right) \right]} \quad (8.12)$

For $x_t = 2 \cdot 5$,

95% c.i. $= 0 \cdot 491 \pm 3 \cdot 182 \sqrt{\left[0 \cdot 0016 \cdot \left(\frac{1}{5} + \frac{(2 \cdot 5 - 3 \cdot 0)^2}{10 \cdot 0} \right) \right]}$

$$= 0 \cdot 431 - 0 \cdot 551.$$

There is a 95% probability that this interval encompasses the mean value $\bar{y}_i$ of the distribution from which the observed value y_i originated. For the example considered $\bar{y}_i$ corresponds to the 'true' optical density.

Answering 8.4, 5.

A 95% c.i. on the observed values Y_i for any given value x_i: say $x_i = 2·5$ as above:

$$95\% \text{ c.i. on } Y_i = Y_i \pm t_{n-2}\sqrt{\left[S_e^2 \cdot \left(1 + \frac{1}{n} + \frac{(x_i - \bar{x})^2}{SS_x} \right) \right]} \quad (8.13)$$

$$= 0·491 \pm 3·182\sqrt{\left[0·0016 \cdot \left(1 + \frac{1}{5} + \frac{(2·5 - 3·0)^2}{10·0} \right) \right]}$$

$$= 0·350\text{--}0·632.$$

There is a 95% probability that, in any repetitions of the readings on this solution, the *observed* optical densities will fall in the range 0·350 to 0·632.

Overall conclusions from the answers to 8.4, 4, and 8.4, 5.

It is important to be quite clear about the distinction between these last two prediction intervals.

If we measure the optical density of a 2·5mg/l calibration solution repeatedly under exactly the same conditions as those of the above experiment, the values recorded will fluctuate between 0·350 and 0·632 (95% of the time). These fluctuations, or measurement errors, are centred around the 'true' optical density of this solution. There is a 95% probability that the interval 0·431 to 0·551 encompasses this 'true' or mean value.

If these prediction intervals are plotted on the graph of $Y = a + b \cdot x$ they exhibit a characteristic shape evident in *Fig. 43*.

Note: From the expressions above it can be deduced that the parameter estimates are improved by:

1. Increasing the total number of observations made (n).

2. Increasing the range over which they are made (SS_x), within the constraints of the straight-line relationship.

3. Reducing the size of the residual variation (S_e^2), by technical improvements in the observation or measurement process, by replication of the measurements at each x_i-value, or by use of supplementary information in a multiple regression analysis (discussed in Chapter 9).

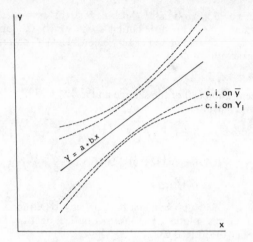

Fig. 43. Prediction intervals for the simple linear regression model.

This information can be usefully employed at the experimental design stage.

8.7. THE CALIBRATION PROBLEM

In the majority of regression experiments in which prediction is an objective, the unknown of interest is the y-variable. Given a new value for the x-variable it is a straightforward matter to produce point and interval estimates for the corresponding y-variable using expressions 8.3, 8.12 and 8.13.

Occasions arise when, given a value y_i, we would like to predict the x-variable (or range of x-variables) from which it arose. This situation is typically represented in the calibration example employed to date. Having estimated the calibration relation between the optical density (y) of a specific analyte and its concentration (x), we will subsequently want to use that calibration line to translate the optical densities recorded for patient's test specimens into concentration values. We assume that the patient's samples have been analyzed in parallel with the standard solutions (calibrators). In this situation it is necessary to invert the regression equation as follows:

$$\text{estimated } \hat{X}_i = y_i - a/b. \qquad (8.14)$$

This is exactly equivalent to 'reading-off' the estimated concentration of a test sample by eye, from a graph of the calibration line. Expression 8.14 is a *non-linear* combination of the random variables a, b and y and as such is subject to a statistical bias: the purely random variation in these variables induces a systematic error in the estimate X_t of purely mathematical origin, i.e. expression 8.14 is not an unbiased estimator of the 'true' concentration of the test specimen. The bias has been estimated approximately by Shukla (1972) for straight-line calibrations:

$$\text{Bias in } \hat{X}_t = \frac{S_e^2 \cdot (\hat{X}_t - \bar{x})}{SS_x \cdot b^2}, \tag{8.15}$$

the terms S_e^2, $\bar{x}$, SS_x and b being derived from the calibration standards, as illustrated in *example 8.2*.

The bias is non-existent at the *calibrator mean* $\bar{x}$. Higher test concentration values are subject to an increasing positive bias (overestimated) whilst lower concentration values are subject to an increasing negative bias.

One immediate result of this observation is that assay methods involving re-calibration with every test batch, with both test samples and calibration standards subject to analytical imprecision, produce results with skewed, i.e. non-Normal, error distributions (*Fig. 44*).

The magnitude of this bias is directly related (from expression 8.15) to the range of the calibrator concentration values (SS_x), the size of the measurement error in the response variable (S_e^2) and the slope of the calibration line (β). For the majority of clinical assays the bias involved will be trivially small, particularly if the foregoing facts are taken into account in designing the assay. It is equally true that the bias is not trivial for some of the less precise assays in use, particularly when dealing with extreme concentration values (low or high), as can be simply demonstrated by substitution of known assay parameters into expression 8.15.

A *prediction interval* for the range of concentration values likely to be associated with any particular response y_t must take into account not only the imprecision of the response variable, but also the uncertainty in the estimated calibration line, which, as we have already seen, leads to some awkward distributional problems for X_t. The problem was addressed by Fieller (1944).

Taken one step at a time, the calculations are straightforward and well within the capacity of a hand-held programmable calculator.

Answering 8.4, 6.

Given an observed optical density (y_i) of 0·90 on a test sample, estimate the concentration (x_i) of the sample and a 95% interval on the range of concentrations likely to give rise to such a reading (using the example of section 8.6).

1. Calculate $A = b^2 - t_{n-2} \cdot S_b^2$, where $S_b^2 = S_e^2/SS_x$

$$A = 0 \cdot 195^2 - (3 \cdot 182 \times 0 \cdot 012\ 65^2)$$
$$= 0 \cdot 037\ 516.$$

2. Calculate

$$B = \frac{t_{n-2}}{A} \cdot \sqrt{\left\{ S_e^2 \cdot \left[A \cdot (1 + \frac{1}{n}) + \frac{(y_i - \bar{y})^2}{SS_x} \right] \right\}}$$

$$B = \frac{3 \cdot 182}{0 \cdot 037\ 516} \cdot \sqrt{\left\{ 0 \cdot 0016 \left[0 \cdot 037\ 516(1 + \frac{1}{5}) + \frac{(0 \cdot 9 - 0 \cdot 588)^2}{10} \right] \right\}}$$

$$= 0 \cdot 793\ 871.$$

3. Calculate the

$$95\% \text{ interval} = \left[\bar{x} + \frac{b \cdot (y_i - \bar{y})}{A} \right] \pm B. \tag{8.16}$$

$$95\% \text{ interval} = \left[3 \cdot 000 + \frac{0 \cdot 195\ (0 \cdot 9 - 0 \cdot 588)}{0 \cdot 037\ 515} \right] \pm 0 \cdot 793\ 871$$

$$= 3 \cdot 83 - 5 \cdot 42.$$

4. Calculate $\hat{X_i} = (y_i - a)/b$.

$$\hat{X_i} = (0 \cdot 9 - 0 \cdot 003)/0 \cdot 195$$
$$= 4 \cdot 60 \text{ units/l.}$$

Conclusions

Our estimate of the test sample concentration is 4·60 with a 95% prediction interval of 3·83 to 5·42.

Note how the interval is asymmetric about the estimate 4.60.

A graphical illustration of the interval is presented in *Fig. 44*. The test sample response y_i has been projected across the graph to the calibration line in order to read-off the corresponding

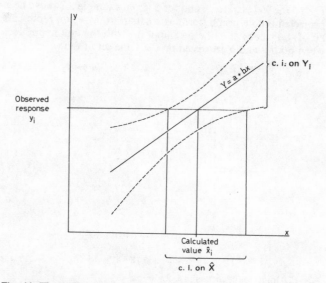

Fig. 44. The calibration problem.

concentration X_t. In so doing, the prediction interval for Y_t constructed about the calibration line using expression 8.13, is cut at two points, which, projected down onto the concentration axis, forms the prediction interval on X_t (given by expression 8.16).

If b is not significantly different from zero, the prediction interval on X_t will be infinite. This is unlikely to prove a practical problem since an assay having such a calibration would not be viable, i.e. if a relationship between the material being assayed and some specific property of that material cannot be established, there is no 'assay'.

8.8. JOINT CONFIDENCE INTERVAL ON α AND β

The 95% c.i. described for α and β are only appropriate for estimation and inference on *one* of the parameters, for any given set of data. If we want to use the 95% c.i. for *both* α and β on the same set of sample data we run into a serious problem, since the 95% c.i. are *not independent* of each other. An example will help to clarify the consequences of this observation. In

Fig. 45 the 95% c.i. for α and for β (from example 8.2) have been projected onto a graph, forming a square; this region represents all of the values of *a* and *b* compatible with the null hypotheses when both *a* and *b* are tested on the same set of data.

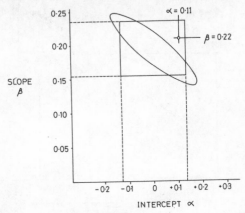

Fig. 45. Joint confidence ellipse for α *and* β.

Suppose that we had started out with the null hypotheses $H_0: \beta = 0 \cdot 22$ *and* $H_0: \alpha = 0 \cdot 11$. Reference to the individual 95% c.i. for α and β would lead to the conclusion that we had insufficient evidence for rejecting either hypothesis. Reference to *Fig. 45* verifies that the joint value defined by these null hypotheses falls within the boxed acceptance region. If we now consider the *joint 95% confidence ellipse* in *Fig. 45*, which takes account of the association between *a* and *b*, we find that the null hypotheses are incompatible with the sample data, i.e. we would reject both null hypotheses, in sharp contrast to the previous conclusion.

The construction of this joint confidence interval is described in detail by its originators Mandel and Linnig (1957).

8.9. THE BIVARIATE NORMAL REGRESSION MODEL

For this model both *x* and *y* are completely uncontrolled (random) variables, drawn from *Normally* distributed populations. The underlying probability model is that of a joint or bivariate Normal distribution. This is somewhat involved mathematically, but it can be visualized on a simple *x–y* graph as a 'cloud' of data points concentrated on the intersection of the x and y means. If the two random variables are independent (*see* Chapter 3) of each other, the points thin out radially from the intersection of the two means, as illustrated in *Fig. 46a*.

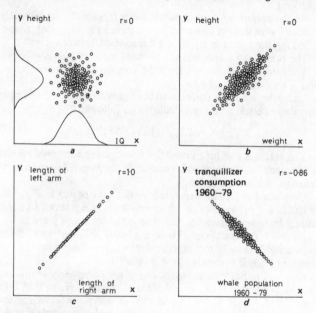

Fig. 46. Patterns of correlation.

In this graph any value of x can be associated with almost any of y. There is no discernible association between the two variables at all.

If the two random variables are related (non-independent), the cloud of data points reflects the degree of association by assuming an elliptical shape as in *Fig. 46b*. If the association between x and y is perfect, so that for any particular value of x there is only one possible value for y, the ellipse collapses onto a perfectly straight line (*Fig. 46c*).

The association may be inverse (or negative) so that high values of x tend to be associated with low values of y, in which case the ellipse appears as in *Fig. 46d*.

The bivariate Normal distribution *parameter* ρ (rho) is a measure of extent to which the two random variables are dependent upon each other. If they are completely independent ρ = 0. If they are perfectly related ρ = 1 (or −1 for a perfect inverse relation).

As the parameter ρ takes values away from zero, the bivariate Normal distribution assumes an increasingly elliptical shape, reflecting the increasingly strong association between x and y.

The parameter ρ is called the *population correlation coefficient*.

The sample statistic r is called the *sample correlation coefficient* and is an estimator of ρ.

Using the summary statistics of the previous section, the sample correlation coefficient r is calculated as follows:

$$r = SS_{xy}/\sqrt{[SS_x \cdot SS_y]} \tag{8.17}$$

The statistic r is an essentially investigative tool used in the assessment of patterns of association between *Normally* distributed random variables.

Consider the picture presented by the data points in *Fig. 46b*. What is the probability of observing a sample pattern like this purely by chance assuming that the variables x and y are in fact unrelated? We could put this in a slightly different way. If the *population* is distributed as *Fig. 46a*, what is the probability of drawing from it a *sample* like *Fig. 46b*?

Our null hypothesis is that x and y are completely unrelated, or independent, i.e. H_0:ρ = 0. Our alternative H_1 is that they are related, i.e. H_1:ρ ≠ 0. To test the null hypothesis we require only the sample correlation coefficient r and the sample size n.

By way of illustration, suppose that $r = 0.300$ and $n = 52$. Refer to Appendix, *Table E*. Locate $n = 50$ in the left hand column and note the critical values of r. At the 5% level the critical value is 0·279 and at the 1% level the critical value is 0·361.

Our test value 0·300 exceeds the 5% value but not the 1% value. The probability of observing the sample value $r = 0.300$ if H_0 were true, i.e. ρ = 0, is between 1:20 and 1:100. This is evidence for rejecting H_0 in favour of H_1, but it is not as strong as we might have wished. It rather depends upon how important it is for you to avoid being wrong.

Remember: the statistic r (Pearson's coefficient of linear correlation) is heavily dependent, for its interpretation, upon the assumption of a bivariate Normal distribution.

You can certainly perform the arithmetic for data such as that in *Fig. 42* (where x has no probability distribution at all) but how exactly you interpret the numbers produced is anyone's guess. Under these sort of conditions the numerical value of r becomes very sensitive to the position of the highest and lowest data points.

Never be tempted to evaluate r without first plotting the data on a graph. In *Fig. 47* the relationship between x and y is quite exact but the linear correlation coefficient r is unlikely to be 1.00, nor anything very near it.

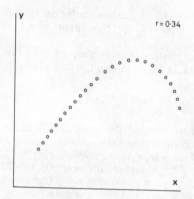

Fig. 47. Non-monotonic curve.

8.10. RANK CORRELATION

Non-parametric measures of association are available for data that do not fit the bivariate Normal model. Kendall's rank correlation coefficient τ and Spearman's rank correlation coefficient r_s are perhaps the best known. Which is the most appropriate in any given situation is not entirely clear. For the purpose of this discussion, Spearman's coefficient has the distinct advantage of being no more than the ordinary correlation coefficient (of expression 8.17) calculated for the *ranks* of the x and y variables. As such, its statistical significance is very easily evaluated using Appendix, *Table E* (for sample sizes $n > 10$).

Example *8.3*

y_t Psychological test score for aggression:	48	26	49	58	72	84	97	36	89	11
x_t Plasma testosterone level in microgm/l:	400	350	650	600	1150	1100	1800	250	1400	100
Rank value of y_1:	4	2	5	6	7	8	10	3	9	1
Rank value of x_t:	4	3	6	5	8	7	10	2	9	1

A straightforward correlation coefficient r, calculated on the rank values, gives us the Spearman correlation coefficient $r_s = 0.964$.

A simpler expression for r_s is given by the following formula, which provides an identical result to that above:

$$r_s = 1 - \frac{6\Sigma d^2}{n(n^2 - 1)}$$

where Σd^2 is the sum of the squared differences between the rank values, and n = sample size (in the example above $n = 10$).

The critical value for r_s is found by entering Appendix, *Table E*, at n, where the 5% value for this example is 0·632 and the 1% value is 0·765. The test value of 0·964 is therefore unlikely to be the product of a purely chance selection from an uncorrelated population. Remember that the 'significant' correlation demonstrated does not imply a causal relationship between testosterone levels and aggression. The result might, however, prompt us to examine the association in the context of a good experimental design.

Spearman's coefficient can be employed on data exhibiting curvature so long as the relationship between x and y is *monotonic*, ie. the curve must not double back on itself as shown in *Fig. 47*.

Correlation coefficients are widely employed in the examination of method comparison data. The assay values for a batch of patient's specimens, established by each of two measurement methods, are compared in order to ascertain how well they agree with each other. The correlation coefficient is of questionable value in this situation and statements to the effect that ' . . . a highly significant correlation ($p < 0.001$) was demonstrated between the results of the two methods' are quite redundant. We already know that the two methods are supposed to be measuring the same thing in the biological samples. If the two sets of results on a common batch of specimens were not significantly correlated, it would be little short of amazing. They do not have to agree particularly well in clinical terms for the essentially non-random structure of this situation to be detected. The real question of interest in the method comparison study is not 'Are the results associated?' but 'Exactly what *form* does the expected association take?' This question is dealt with in Chapter 10.

8.11. PREDICTION FROM THE BIVARIATE REGRESSION MODEL

For the simple linear regression model we had only one regression line that made any logical sense, that of $Y = a + bx + e$. We could use this estimated regression equation to predict the likely value of y, given a value for x. For example, if x was the dose of a drug administered to a patient and y was the subsequent elevation in the subject's blood pressure, it would be perfectly reasonable to use the regression equation to predict the likely blood pressure given some intermediate value for the drug dose. The simple linear model reflects our belief that the elevation in blood pressure is, to some extent, determined by the dose of drug administered. Reversing the prediction process to predict x, given a value for y, would make little sense. Blood pressure levels do not determine the dose of drug administered.

Occasions arise when a reverse prediction might be required as evidenced in the case of calibration relationships, dealt with in section 8.7, in which case we invert the regression equation:

$$\text{predicted } \hat{X}_t = (y_t - a)/b. \qquad (8.18)$$

For the bivariate model we have no formal assumptions about the nature of the association between x and y. Indeed, our null-hypothesis is that there is no association between them. Both variables are random and the question put to them is essentially exploratory: ' ... is there evidence in the sample data for a statistically significant association between the two random variables?' *If* there is, we can set about the formation of a hypothesis as to the nature of the association, and then design an experiment to test that hypothesis within the framework of a simple linear regression model.

Alternatively, we may not be interested in the structure of the association as such (indeed it may resist exact definition), in which case our interest might be confined to using what association there is in a quite empirical manner for predicting the likely value of one variable given a value for the other. Since *both* variables are quite random, the model is symmetrical, i.e. we could just well use x to predict y, as we could use y to predict x.

For the *prediction of y*, we use the regression of y on x, employing expressions 8.7 and 8.8 for the slope b and the intercept a.

$$Y = a + b \cdot x + e.$$

This equation is formed by minimizing the y-residuals from the fitted line. A 95% c.i. for the predicted value of y is obtained directly from expression 8.13.

For the *prediction of x*, we use the regression of x on y:

$$X = \acute{a} + \acute{b} \cdot y + e.$$

This equation is formed by minimizing the x-residuals from the fitted line, in sharp contrast to the procedure adopted in expression 8.18 for predicting x in the simple linear model.

Note: Slope $\acute{b} = SS_{xy}/SS_y$
            Intercept $\acute{a} = \bar{x} - b \cdot \bar{y}$

95% c.i. on predicted $\hat{X}_i$

$$= \hat{X}_i \pm t_{n-2} \cdot \sqrt{\left\{ S_e{}^2 \cdot \left[1 + \frac{1}{n} + \frac{(y_i - \bar{y})^2}{SS_y} \right] \right\}}$$

where $S_e{}^2 = [SS_x - (SS_{xy})^2/SS_y]/(n-2)$.

Note: A significant association between x and y could be deduced from a test of the null hypothesis $H_0: \beta = 0$, using the 95% c.i. described for the simple linear regression model (expression 8.10). The regression approach has a considerable advantage over the correlation coefficient r in that we are also provided with valuable additional information in the form of a prediction equation and intervals, should the association prove significant.

It is useful to note that the two regression lines of the bivariate model cross each other at a point on the graph defined by $\bar{x}$ and $\bar{y}$. When the variables x and y are perfectly associated (*Fig. 46c*) the two lines are identically superimposed. When the two variables are completely independent of each other (*Fig. 46a*), the two lines cross each other at right angles, the regression line $Y = a + b \cdot x$ being parallel to the x-axis, i.e. $\beta = 0$.

Errors of measurement in the x variable that would have seriously disturbed the simple linear regression model are entirely acceptable in the bivariate model. For this latter model we are interested in the *observed* variation. We take the x and y variables entirely at face value.

8.12. BEYOND THE LOOKING-GLASS

A sharp distinction has been drawn between the simple and bivariate regression models. For the simple model we control or fix x, and observe the response (random) y. For the bivariate model both x and y are random.

Implicit in our discussion of the simple model has been this idea of controlling the x variable, selecting specific values at which we can observe the corresponding variable y. If it is *known* that the relationship to be studied satisfies the assumptions of the simple linear model, it is quite possible to take values of x at random, but treat them as if they were fixed by the experimenter. The 'distribution' of the x values does not have to conform to any particular type.

Note: This generalization of the simple linear model must be carefully distinguished from the bivariate model, since x and y now appear to be random in both models.

The simple model continues to assume that a quite specific form of relationship exists within the experimental framework employed, i.e. the x variable (free of measurement error) will be exactly related to the means of the corresponding y variables. The relation may be the product of a scientific law or law-like process in which the variable x determines the mean response y, and as such is uniquely described by only one regression line $Y = a + b \cdot x$.

The bivariate model makes no such assumptions. It is primarily investigative, being used to establish whether a significant association exists at all between two normally distributed random variables x and y. If an association is established, it can be used as a basis for quite empirical predictions on either variable, for which two regression lines of a purely predictive nature can be conceived. The nature of the association remains undefined.

REFERENCES

Anscombe F. J. (1973) Graphs in statistical analysis. *Am. Statistician* **27,** 17–21.

Armitage P. (1974) *Statistical Methods in Medical Research*. Oxford, Blackwell.

Berkson J. (1950) Are there two regressions? *J. Am. Statist. Ass.* **45,** 164–180.

Fieller E. C. (1944) A fundamental formula in the statistics of biological assay and some applications. *Q. J. Pharm.* **17,** 117–123.

Healy M. J. R. (1968) The disciplining of medical data. *Br. Med. Bull.* **24,** 210–214.

Mandel J. (1964) *The Statistical Analysis of Experimental Data*. New York, Wiley.

Mandel J. and Linnig F. J. (1957) Study of accuracy in chemical analysis using linear calibration curves. *An. Chem.* **29,** 743–749.

Neave H. R. (1978) *Statistical Tables*. London, Allen & Unwin.

Shukla G. K. (1972) On the problem of calibration. *Technometrics* **14,** 547–553.

Snedecor G. W. and Cochran W. G. (1974) *Statistical Methods*. Ames, Iowa State Univ.

9 Multivariate Analysis

In the previous chapter we considered in some detail the analysis of relationships involving two variables, in the context of what might be called a fixed model (the simple linear regression) or a random model (the bivariate regression). Multivariate analysis extends the consideration to three or more variables.

The analyses may be investigative, seeking out patterns or regularities in large bodies of data, or they may be directed towards the comparison of large or complex groups of data, identifying their points of similarity or dissimilarity. The analyses may be based upon quite complex multivariate statistical models; they may be quite empirical. The techniques used are a blend of mathematical statistics, the calculus, geometry and algebra— the computer being an essential working tool.

We will do little more than extend the regression models of the previous chapter into the shallows of multivariate analysis, far enough to sample some of their possibilities and limitations.

9.1. REGRESSION REVISITED

In the previous chapter one of the objectives of a regression analysis was the use of one variable to predict the value of another. It may be that the observation of a variable y is difficult and/or expensive whilst the variable x is correspondingly cheap or simple to obtain. If a significant relationship exists between x and y (i.e. $\beta \neq 0$) both statistically and practically, we can save ourselves a good deal of trouble by measuring x and using it to predict the probable value of y.

If we examine the nature of this prediction process just a little more carefully it will simplify the extension to multivariate regression analysis which underpins several branches of multivariate analysis and for which a *simple* graphical explanation is difficult to achieve.

We have a random variable y, let us say an index of aggression, obtained from a psychometric test profile. We will assume this variable to be Normally distributed in the population under study.

153

Suppose that we now select a subject at random from this same population, but instead of measuring his aggression index we measure another variable, the plasma testosterone level (x) which we will also assume to be a *Normally* distributed variable. Can this information be used to tell us anything very useful about the subject's likely aggression index?

1. If x is completely unrelated to y a graph of the paired measurements in a random sample of subjects from the population might look something like *Fig. 48*.

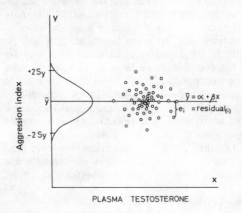

PLASMA TESTOSTERONE

Fig. 48. Independent variables ($\beta = 0$).

A least-squares regression line $Y = a + bx + e$ would be horizontal to the x-axis, i.e. it would have a population slope $\beta = 0$ and an intercept of $\bar{y}$.

The variable x in this situation tells us absolutely nothing at all about the likely value of y. In calculating the least-squares line we minimized the squared y_i residuals (e in *Fig. 49*) about the fitted line. The overall variation of the y_i values about the line is conveniently summarized by the variance of the residuals, S_e^2. (We use the variance since it has rather more useful mathematical properties than its square-root, the standard deviation.)

The residual variation of the data points about the calculated line in *Fig. 48* is at a maximum and will be identical to the total variation in y, S_y^2 (equivalent to the 'residual' variation about $\bar{y}$).

2. If the plasma testosterone levels are related to the aggression index, the regression line will have a slope that is significantly different from zero. The residual variation about the fitted line S_e^2 will be significantly smaller than the residual variation about the mean $\bar{y}$. *Figs. 49a* and *49b* illustrate this conclusion.

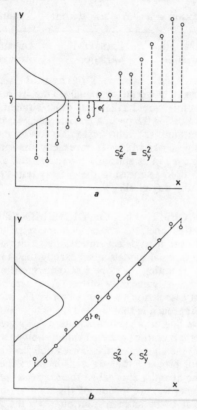

Fig. 49a. Residual variation about the mean y.

    b. Residual variation about the adjusted mean $y = \alpha + \beta x$.

This observation forms the basis of the test of the null hypothesis H_0: $\beta = 0$ in Chapter 8. *If the residual variance S_e^2 is significantly smaller than the total variance of y, S_y^2, the slope $\beta \neq 0$.*

We could now argue that the inclusion of the x variable in the regression equation has explained some of the variation in y:

$$\underbrace{Y}_{} = \underbrace{a + bx}_{} + \underbrace{e}_{}$$

$$\underbrace{\text{Aggression}}_{\substack{\text{Total} \\ \text{variation}}} = \underbrace{a + b \cdot \overset{\text{Plasma}}{\text{testosterone}}}_{\substack{\text{Explained} \\ \text{variation}}} + \underbrace{\text{Residual}}_{\substack{\text{Unexplained} \\ \text{variation}}} \quad (9.1)$$

Taken to a logical extreme, if the residual e were zero, all of the variation in y would be explained by its regression on x. The data points would fall in an exact straight line. Given a particular value for the plasma testosterone, we could state with complete certainty the value of the aggression index, assuming that the subject was drawn from exactly the same population as that employed in establishing the values of a and b, and that the method used to measure the plasma testosterone had not changed in any way at all.

9.2. THE COEFFICIENT OF DETERMINATION
The correlation coefficient r is in many respects a redundant statistic. We use it to detect statistically significant associations in bivariate Normal models when exactly the same information is provided by testing the slope b of the regression $Y = a + bx$, i.e. is the slope b significantly different from zero? If it is, there is a significant association between x and y. The advantage of the regression approach is that we end up with a lot more besides; a descriptive line, a prediction equation for y given x and confidence intervals on the predicted values should they be required.

However, the square of the correlation coefficient r^2 has a rather useful property that we can tie in to the previous discussion. The quantity r^2 is called the *coefficient of determination* and represents the proportion of the total variation in y that can be explained by its regression on x. By the same argument the quantity $1 - r^2$ is the proportion of the variation in y that remains unexplained, this making up the residual e.

9.3. MULTIPLE REGRESSION
In the prediction equation $Y = a + bx + e$, the variable x is commonly referred to as an independent variable. We will use

the descriptive term 'explanatory variable'. If a knowledge of plasma testosterone levels explains some of the variation in the aggression index we could use the equation $Y = a + bx + e$ to predict aggression. There would be some uncertainty in the prediction reflected in the size of the residual e, the unexplained variation.

Suppose that, in addition to the plasma testosterone measurement we had also recorded the patient's systolic blood pressure, which we also believe to be related to the aggression index. Is there any way we could use this additional information to improve our prediction still further?

We can utilize the multiple linear regression model of expression 9.2,

$$y = \alpha + \beta_1 x_1 + \beta_2 x_2 + \varepsilon \tag{9.2}$$

where x_1 = plasma testosterone concentration in ng/ml
and x_2 = systolic blood pressure in mm Hg.

Instead of a regression line on a two dimensional surface (the x–y graph), we now have a regression plane in the three dimensional graph space. The residuals ε are the distances of the observed data points (each defined in the graph space by values for y, x_1 and x_2) from the fitted regression plane. This plane is fitted by least-squares, i.e. it minimizes the squared residuals of the data points from the regression plane.

The most important assumptions for the multiple regression model are independent, Normally distributed residuals with a constant variance.

In practice we would be obliged to estimate the parameters of expression 9.2 from a random sample, giving us the estimated equation 9.3,

$$Y = a + b_1 x_1 + b_2 x_2 + e. \tag{9.3}$$

The coefficients b_1 and b_2 are called partial regression coefficients. If we calculate the multivariate regression equation with both plasma testosterone levels and systolic blood pressure measurements we can assess the usefulness of the blood pressure variable from the size of the residual e in 9.3. If the estimated residual variance is significantly smaller than that from the regression on testosterone levels alone, we have some evidence for the value of blood pressure measurements in improving the aggression index prediction. The statistical test used to compare the residual variances is the variance ratio or F-test, described in detail in Snedecor and Cochran (1974).

This line of reasoning extends to the use of three, four or forty explanatory variables. The regression plane becomes rather abstract, a hyperplane in the multidimensional vector space, but little is lost by leaving this complication to the mathematics.

Stepwise regression methods examine large numbers of explanatory variables, regressing them in a variety of combinations on y, seeking out the subset which gives the maximum reduction in the residual variance. Since every additional explanatory variable used in the equation demands time and money for its collection, the pursuit of optimal, efficient prediction equations is of real importance. The multiple linear regression model is one of the more important working tools of applied statistics. Ovid passed the apt comment 'Things worthless singly are often useful collectively'.

It is possible to calculate a *multiple correlation coefficient R*, (generally provided as a part of the multiple regression program output on a computer) and the quantity R^2 is interpreted in exactly the same way as r^2, the coefficient of determination. It is the proportion of the variation in y that can be explained by the regression on the explanatory variables.

Having calculated a multiple regression equation, do not for a moment forget that it is only validly employed for prediction using measurements obtained in exactly the same way as those of the original sample. If you change your plasma testosterone assay from a radioimmunoassay to a cytochemical bioassay, the multiplier b_1 in expression 9.3 is no longer appropriate.

Remember also that the prediction is only valid for subjects drawn from the original population studied.

9.4. LINEAR DISCRIMINANT ANALYSIS

Suppose that the aggression index of the previous example had provided nothing more than a categorical statement of whether the subject was aggressive or passive. If the results of the test scored $y = 1$ for an aggressive result and $y = 0$ for a passive result, a straightforward multiple regression of x_1 (plasma testosterone ng/ml) and x_2 (systolic blood pressure mm Hg) on y, using the results from a suitable random sample of test subjects, would provide a prediction equation of the form:

$$Y = a + b_1x_1 + b_2x_2$$

If we discard the 'intercept' term a we are left with a linear discriminant function Z:

$$Z = b_1x_1 + b_2x_2 \qquad (9.4)$$

The practical use of this function is suggested in *Fig. 50*. For both the aggressive and the passive groups there is a marked overlap in the observed plasma testosterone and blood pressure measurements. As they stand it would not be easy to allocate a new test subject to any particular group simply on the basis of these two measurements. The linear discriminant function Z is the linear combination of the x variables that best separates (or discriminates between) the two groups. For two x variables, the geometrical interpretation of Z is a straight line separation of the two-dimensional group ellipses.

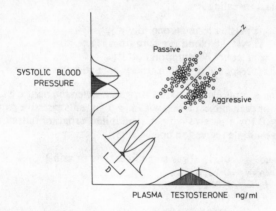

Fig. 50. Discrimination between two patient groups on the basis of two measured variables.

If three variables are used the data points are defined in three-dimensions, the elliptical classification groups of *Fig. 50* becoming three-dimensional ellipsoids, clouds of points in the graph space:

$$Z = b_1x_1 + b_2x_2 + b_3x_3 \qquad (9.5)$$

The linear discriminant function Z is now a flat plane separating the ellipsoids. Four or more variables define hyperellipsoids in a multidimensional graph space. The function Z now describes a hyperplane which is conceptually difficult to grasp, but in the form of equation 9.6 is a simple enough extension of its predecessors:

$$Z = b_1x_1 + b_2x_2 + b_3x_3 + \ldots + b_nx_n \qquad (9.6)$$

Example

Suppose that we have a sample of fifty patients, of whom thirty are known to be aggressive and twenty are known to be passive. This knowledge might be derived from their 'aggression index' scores; it might be derived from long-term sociological/criminological observation.

On each of the fifty subjects we measure a number of variables, say four, which in isolation are not sufficient to indicate the aggressive status of the subject, but which taken together may provide a revealing insight:

x_1: plasma testosterone (ng/ml);
x_2: systolic blood pressure (mm Hg);
x_3: alcohol consumption (g/d);
x_4: response time to artificial pain stimulus (s).

Using a multiple regression program, enter the values x_1, x_2, x_3, x_4 for each subject along with $y = 1$ for an aggressive patient or $y = 0$ for a passive patient. The initial program output will be the multiple regression coefficients:

$a = 0.63;$ (a is sometimes written as b_0)
$b_1 = 0.10;$
$b_2 = -0.002;$
$b_3 = 0.05;$
$b_4 = -0.08.$

Discard the intercept a. The remaining coefficients make up the discriminant function Z:

$$Z = 0.10x_1 - 0.002x_2 + 0.05x_3 - 0.08x_4$$

Table 14 presents the means of each of the variables observed for the aggressive and passive groups, and for the combined groups.

MULTIVARIATE ANALYSIS 161

Table 14

	n	mean x_1	mean x_2	mean x_3	mean x_4
Aggressive subjects (A)	30	11·5	118	75	7
Passive subjects (P)	20	4·5	136	5	11
Means $\frac{1}{2}(A + P)$		8·0	127	40	9

The centroids of the aggressive and passive groups are obtained by substitution of the aggressive and passive group means into the discriminant equation:

Aggressive group centroid
$$= (0·1·11·5) - (0·002·118) + (0·05·75) - (0·08·7) = 4·104;$$
Passive group centroid
$$= (0·1·4·5) - (0·002·136) + (0·05·5) - (0·08·11) = -0·452.$$

The midway point between the two group centroids, $Z_0 = [4·104 + (-0·452)]/2 = 1·826$, is a convenient cut-off point for the allocation of new test subjects.

If we now measure the four variables in a new test subject drawn from exactly the same population as that of the original sample group, using exactly the same measurement techniques, we can employ the calculated discriminant Z to allocate the subject to the most appropriate group. If Z exceeds Z_0 the subject is classified as aggressive; if Z is less than Z_0 the subject is classified as passive.

The procedure is somewhat simplified by shifting Z_0 to zero, in this case by subtracting Z_0 (1·826) from Z:

$$Z = (0·10x_1 - 0·002x_2 + 0·05x_3 - 0·08x_4) - 1·826.$$

By setting Z_0 to zero we need only consider the sign of Z, rather than its value relative to Z_0, e.g.

new subject: $x_1 = 12·0$ ng/ml,
$$x_2 = 110 \text{ mm Hg},$$
$$x_3 = 52·5 \text{ g/d},$$
$$x_4 = 5·31 \text{ s};$$
$$Z = (0·10·12·0) - (0·002·110) + (0·05·52·5)$$
$$- (0·08·31) - 1·826$$
$$= +1·354.$$

The positive value of Z suggests an allocation to the aggressive group.

9.5. EFFECTIVENESS OF ALLOCATION .

The effectiveness of the allocation procedure can be expressed directly in terms of the proportion of new subjects who would be correctly classified on the basis of the calculated discriminant function.

One rather appealing way of determining this is to use the discriminant function on every one of the fifty subjects in the original test sample. We already know which of these are aggressive and which are passive. If the discriminant function identifies twenty-eight of the thirty aggressive subjects correctly, it is, on the basis of the evidence available, 93% effective. This is an optimistic estimate and unreliable for small sample sizes.

Another widely used measure employs an important quantity known as the *Mahalanobis generalized distance*, D. This is a standardized measure of the 'distance' between the two group centroids expressed in terms of standard deviations.

A centroid is the central point of a multivariate ellipsoid or hyperellipsoid. It can be visualized as the multivariate equivalent of a mean, the 'central' point of a symmetrical univariate distribution.

If $D = 0$ the two ellipsoids are identically superimposed, no discrimination at all being possible. If D is greater than 4, the centroids are more than four standard deviations apart, the overlap between the two ellipsoids along the discriminant plane being correspondingly small.

There are several ways of calculating D. If a multiple regression program has been used, part of the computer output can be conveniently employed for this purpose. To understand the origins of the numbers we require, it is necessary to break down the multiple regression equation as follows in expression 9.7 (this being a logical extension of the linear regression breakdown of expression 9.1).

$$\underbrace{Y}_{\substack{\text{Total} \\ \text{variation} \\ \text{(Total } SS)}} = \underbrace{b_0 + b_1x_1 + b_2x_2 + \ldots b_nx_n +}_{\substack{\text{Explained} \\ \text{variation} \\ \text{(Regression } SS)}} \underbrace{e}_{\substack{\text{Unexplained} \\ \text{variation} \\ \text{(Residual } SS)}} \quad (9.7)$$

The multiple regression of $x_1, x_2 \ldots x_n$ on y seeks to explain the variation in y (the thing we are really interested in!) in terms of the x variables. A good multiple regression program will deliver as a part of its output an analysis of variance (ANOVA), partitioning the total variance of y into that *explained* by its regression on the x-variables (the regression sum of squares; *Regression SS*) and that which remains unexplained, the *Residual SS*.

For our example problem the relevant part of the ANOVA output is as follows:

ANOVA of multiple regression

Source	SS
Regression	12·93
Residual	5·07
Total	18·00

Mahalanobis generalized D distance

$$= \sqrt{\left[\frac{(n_1 + n_2)\cdot(n_1 + n_2 - 2)}{n_1 \cdot n_2} \cdot \frac{\text{regression } SS}{\text{residual } SS}\right]} \quad (9.8)$$

$$= \sqrt{\left[\frac{(30 + 20)(30 + 20 - 2)}{30 \cdot 20} \cdot \frac{12\cdot93}{5\cdot07}\right]}$$

$$= 3\cdot19.$$

An approximate interpretation of the effectiveness of the discrimination can be obtained by locating $D/2$ in the tables of the Normal probability integral (Appendix, *Table B*) e.g. $D/2 = 1\cdot60$. Locate $1\cdot6$ in the left-hand column and read across to 0. The tabulated integral is $0\cdot4452$. Add $0\cdot5$ to this value. The overall cumulative probability of correct allocation is therefore $0\cdot9452$ or $94\cdot5\%$. This technique makes some stringent assumptions about the statistical properties of the model which will be discussed a little later on; it also tends to provide an optimistic estimate.

More reliable assessments of the discriminant effectiveness employ what are called *jackknife* estimates, but these really do require a computer to handle the laborious calculations involved.

A useful extension of the discriminant function is the recalculation of the %-effectiveness with subsets of the x-variables.

Variables	%-effectiveness of discrimination
$x_1\ x_2\ x_3\ x_4$	94·5%
$x_1\ x_2\ x_3$	89·2%
$x_1\ x_2\ x_4$	94·35%

Only two subsets are shown by way of illustration. The pain response time, x_4, contributes 5·3% to the discrimination whilst x_3, the alcohol consumption, contributes only 0·15%, hardly enough to justify its retention. We can do almost as well without it!

The linear discriminant function is really beginning to reveal its potential in unravelling just how important individual variables are in the decision making process. By calculating the efficiency of a discriminant for a particular disease state with different combinations of laboratory tests, optimal test profiles can be identified. If a particular assay is found to contribute very little to the discrimination it can be discontinued, saving the laboratory time and money.

9.6. MODIFYING THE ALLOCATION CUT-OFF

The cut-off point Z_0 was set at the mid-point between the group centroids. As such, it assumes the population to have equal numbers of aggressive and passive subjects. *If* our base sample of 50 subjects was an unbiased (random) sample from the population of interest we might take the 30: 20 ratio of aggressive to passive subjects to be typical of the population as a whole. If this is the case, the cut-off point Z_0 should be shifted from the mid-point towards the smaller group by the amount $\log_e W/D$ where W = ratio of the larger to the smaller group; e.g., for the aggression study

$$W = 30/20 = 1·5,$$

therefore $\log_e W/D = \log_e 1·5/3·19 = 0·127$.

The original value for Z_0 was 1·826. We shift it towards the passive centroid ($-0·452$) by subtracting 0·127. Modified $Z_0 = 1·699$.

9.7. ASSUMPTIONS FOR THE LINEAR DISCRIMINANT FUNCTION

The calculation of the discriminant function assumes that the ellipses of *Figure 50*, or their multidimensional analogues (ellipsoids and hyperellipsoids), have the same size and shape with the same orientation of their axes on the graph (or in the graph space). *Figure 51a* represents these assumptions graphically for the two-variable case. The size assumption is perhaps the most flexible, *Fig. 51b* being acceptable for many purposes. *Figures 51c* and *51d* represent unacceptable failures of the (homogeneity) assumptions for orientation and shape respectively. A quadratic discriminant function would be appropriate to this more complicated situation.

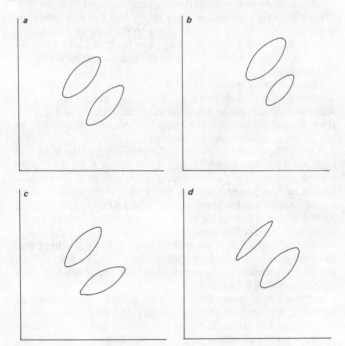

Fig. 51. Size, shape and orientation of discriminant groups for the two-variable case. *Fig. a* represents the distributional requirements for the *linear* discriminant function.

The *homogeneity assumption* is the subject of specific statistical tests for which reference to the specialist literature should be made.

Transformations of the x-variable(s) may be employed to obtain a more satisfactory approximation of the required model, although the overall effects of any transformation must be carefully considered.

For the multiple regression relation the distributional assumption is that the x's are fixed quantities and that y is Normally distributed about a mean given by expression 9.2. In discriminant analysis, the assumption is that y is an indicator variable distinguishing the two groups, while within each group the x's have a multivariate Normal distribution.

Considerable liberties are often taken with the x-variables, to the extent of reducing some of them to dichotomous variables, e.g. smoker, $x = 1$; non-smoker, $x = 0$. This leads to some complicated disturbances in the model and should be left to the statistician.

The Mahalanobis generalized distance D is directly related to another statistic, Hotelling's T^2, which can be used to test the statistical significance of the separation between the two groups. Both D and T^2 assume a *multivariate Normal distribution*, in addition to the homogeneity assumption.

It would be unwise to minimize the complexity of the analytical methods now being considered. In Chapter 3 we had quite enough trouble simply validating the use of a Normal approximation. The homework required for a discriminant analysis to realise its considerable potential is a good deal more complicated. The computer will provide you with a set of discriminant coefficients for the first hundred numbers in a telephone directory; it isn't fussy about the data it works upon. The only thing that has changed about the old truism 'rubbish-in, rubbish-out' since the microprocessor revolution is that now the rubbish is produced a good deal faster.

Allocations to more than just two groups, the province of canonical discriminant analysis, extends the 'diagnostic range' of the discriminant principle. Instead of asking whether a particular laboratory/clinical profile suggests liver disease or no, we can now consider a partition into several clinical categories of liver disease, with the same potential for identifying optimal test profiles.

An excellent review and extensive bibliography of discriminant analysis is available by Solberg (1978).

9.8. IS THERE A PATTERN?
The methods described to date have all assumed a structure in the data (approximated by the statistical model). This has been

utilized in the analyses to inquire further into the structure itself or to make qualified predictions.

A whole area of multivariate analysis is devoted to seeking out structure in the first place. Is there a pattern in the observed results, or underlying the observed results? If there is, can it be used to reduce or summarize the most important properties of the data? Does it give us any insight into the mechanisms by which the results were generated?

The two best known techniques in this area are perhaps Cluster analysis and Factor analysis. Cluster analysis is an important working tool of the Taxonomist seeking out points of similarity and dissimilarity between classes of individuals as a basis for taxonomic classification.

Factor analysis does assume a model for the data, but one that is very much at the command of the analyst. It seeks to explain the variation in complex bodies of data in terms of specific hypothetical 'factors' and the techniques have been applied widely in psychology and the social sciences. The method comes in for some criticism, largely directed at the reality of these 'factors', on the grounds that different analysts can have different views about the nature and number of factors required and thereby proceed to different analytical conclusions with the same body of data.

9.9. CURVATURE

Before leaving the multivariate regression model it is worth noting one more practical application to which it lends itself, unrelated to the previous discussion.

Occasions often arise when we are obliged to deal with relationships that do not conform to the straight-line model. Sometimes the curvature assumes a well-defined functional form that can be converted to a straight-line by transformation of one or both variables involved.

For example, if a percentage change in y is directly related to a constant change in x, we have a curved relationship of the form $y = ae^{bx}$, where a and b are the constants and e is the base of the natural logarithm. If we plot log y against x we obtain a straight line of the form log $y = \log a + b (\log_e)x$, illustrated in *Fig. 52*.

A word of caution about the residual variance, which is assumed to be *constant* throughout the measurement range for the regression models. *If* the variance increases proportionally with the absolute value of y, the logarithmic transformation of y not only linearizes the relationship, but stabilizes the residual variance as well, as shown in *Fig. 52*. This is an extremely useful property of the logarithmic transformation, but it is worth considering its effect upon the residual variance when it happens to be constant in the original data.

The following procedure for determining the nature of a curved relationship is adapted from Natrella (1963), and is summarized in *Table 15*.

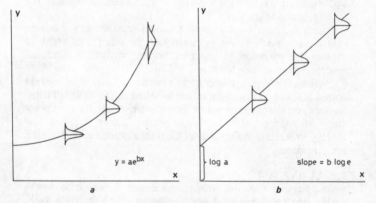

Fig. 52. An example of a linearizing transformation.

1. Plot y against $1/x$ using ordinary graph paper. If a straight-line is obtained the relationship is $y = a + b/x$.

2. Plot $1/y$ against x using ordinary graph paper. If a straight-line is obtained the relationship is either $y = 1/(a + bx)$ or $1/y = a + bx$.

3. Using *semi-log* paper plot x on the arithmetic scale and y on the log-scale. If a straight-line is obtained the relationship is either $y = ae^{bx}$ or $y = ab^x$.

4. Using *log–log* paper plot x against y. If a straight line is obtained the relationship is $y = ax^b$.

Table 15.

Relationship	Calculate straight-line regression $Y_0 = a_0 + b_0 x_0$		Convert a_0 and b_0 to constants a and b	
	x_0	y_0	a_0	b_0
$y = a + b/x$	$1/x$	y	a	b
$y = 1/(a + bx)$ $1/y = a + bx$ $\Big\}$	x	$1/y$	a	b
$y = ae^{bx}$	x	$\log y$	$\log a$	$b \log_e$
$y = ab^x$	x	$\log y$	$\log a$	$\log b$
$y = ax^b$	$\log x$	$\log y$	$\log a$	b

If the curvature resists these functional approximations, a polynomial approximation may be found satisfactory:

linear: $\quad Y = a + bx$;

quadratic: $\quad Y = a + b_1 x + b_2 x^2$;

cubic: $\quad Y = a + b_1 x + b_2 x^2 + b_3 x^3$;

quartic: $\quad Y = a + b_1 x + b_2 x^2 + b_3 x^3 + b_4 x^4$. $\quad$ (9.9)

These expressions are linear in their coefficients b_i. The curves they describe are illustrated in *Fig. 53*.

Polynomial curves must be treated with care. They describe curves of the form illustrated in *Fig. 53* and, when applied to a given set of data, they will attempt to describe them as best they can (in a least-squares sense) by such a curve. If the number of data points on the graph is one more than the *degree* of the polynomial (the number of coefficients b_i) it will fit the points exactly. This leads to the risk of 'overfitting' the data. *Fig. 54a* shows three data points observed on what is in fact a straight-line relation, the deviation of the points from the line being attributable to random variation in y. A quadratic curve fitted to the points in *Fig. 54b* describes them exactly. We would be unwise to draw any dramatic conclusions from this observation. The quadratic curve is obliged to fit exactly any three points in two dimensions!

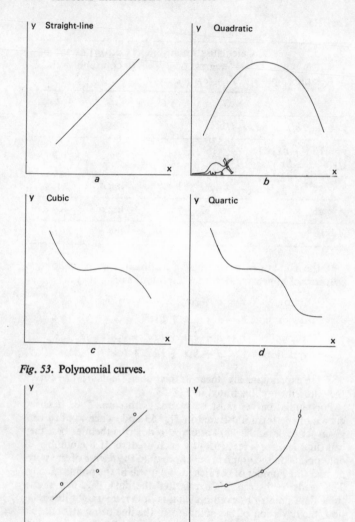

Fig. 53. Polynomial curves.

Fig. 54. Overfitting sample data.

A second caution concerns the use of calculated polynomial equations for making predictions about the value of y beyond the range of the observed points. Polynomials may be visualized as flexible steel wires of particular shapes. They can be bent to a certain extent to meet our needs but all they really want to do is spring back into their original shape. The data points on a graph constrain the polynomial in a similar way, and beyond the constraint of those data points the polynomial 'springs back', in a manner of speaking, to its natural form. This can be extreme for high-order polynomials making even the slightest extrapolation very risky indeed.

Polynomial functions can be treated as a special case of multiple regression, the powers of x being 'explanatory' variables:

$$x_1 = x$$
$$x_2 = x^2$$
$$x_3 = x^3 \text{ etc.}$$

The multiple regression equations take the form shown in expression 9.9. The residual e, the 'unexplained' variation in y, can now be used to assess the goodness-of-fit of the polynomial. If the residual about a straight-line is significantly reduced by fitting a quadratic, but no further reduction is observed for a cubic fit, it might be concluded that a quadratic curve most adequately described the data. This assumes that there are more than enough data points to avoid the trap of overfitting. Remember, sixteen data points would be perfectly described by a fifteenth degree polynomial. This is hardly strong evidence for the existence of a real scientific relationship of such complexity!

If the curvature is complex and we do not wish to run the risks involved in fitting high-order polynomials which can become mathematically ill-behaved, we may resort to a Spline approximation. This procedure splits the curve into segments, each described by a low-order polynomial (cubic) with a clever mathematical device for smoothing out the joins between each polynomial piece, so that the overall curve is smooth. The multiple regression model can yet again accommodate this sophistication although numerical methods are more widely employed.

Non-linear regression problems are discussed in Snedecor and Cochran (1974).

REFERENCES

Natrella M. G. (1963) *Experimental Statistics. NBS Handbook 91.* Washington D.C., *U.S. Govt. Printing Office.*

Snedecor G. W. and Cochran W. G. (1974) *Statistical Methods.* Ames, Iowa State Univ.

Solberg H. E. (1978) Discriminant analysis. *CRC Crit. Rev. in Clin. Lab. Sci.* Nov. 209–242.

10 Method Comparison Studies

'Comparison is the expedient of those who cannot reach the heart of the things compared.' G. Santayana.

It is not uncommon for the clinical laboratory to be tasked with the examination and evaluation of new assay methods or 'test-kits'. Amongst the many technical and economic points that might be considered will be the degree of correspondence between the results produced by the new assay method and those of a 'reference' method. Do the two methods produce, on average, the same results for the same test specimens? The question is an important one. Systematic disagreement between the results of the two assay methods compared can be interpreted in two fundamentally different ways depending upon the assumptions made for the reference method.

10.1. A STUDY IN ACCURACY

Suppose that the new method is in fact a newly-developed chemistry, and as a part of the general assessment of the method we would like some insight into its accuracy. Does the assay-method in fact measure exactly what we want it to measure, no more, no less?

Accuracy might be defined as '... the agreement between the estimate of a quality and its true value'. A given biological sample undoubtedly has some definite amount of the material of interest in it (in a gravimetric sense) at any given point in time. However, our only access to this quantity, the absolute true value, is through measurement. The measurement process is subject to a number of rigorous assumptions (Jerne and Wood, 1949) the validity of some of which can never be established beyond doubt. This may be compounded in the clinical laboratory by the complexity of the test sample's composition and an often incomplete knowledge of the structure, state and behaviour of the material under assay. Whatever the exact case, we can never know in any absolute sense the 'true value' of a biological sample; this applies just as much to the measurement of serum sodium concentration as it does to the measurement of para-thyroid hormone.

Despite the ultimate uncertainty, accuracy remains an ideal well worth the pursuit. The closer that different laboratories (with different assay principles) get to measuring the same thing, the better must be their agreement with each other with clear benefits for the communication of information from one source to another for diagnostic purposes. Accuracy may be an abstraction, but it is good for patients.

Progress is achieved by adopting a consensus view of accuracy. Theoretical considerations, technical knowledge and such clinical experience as is available are used as a basis for selecting one particular method of measurement as a definitive method for the particular substance of interest. It is the most accurate method available in the sense that it best reflects the truth insofar as it is known.

The International Federation of Clinical Chemistry (IFCC, 1979) have recommended the following definition for the *definitive method:* 'A method which after exhaustive investigation is found to have no known source of inaccuracy or ambiguity. The result is termed definitive and is the best known approximation to the true value'.

The National Bureau of Standards (NBS) in the United States have been very active in establishing such methods for a number of the simpler clinical analytes such as sodium, potassium, chloride, calcium, iron, to name but a few. For calcium the estimated uncertainty of a definitive assay result is in the region of 0.1%. The methods are extremely specialized, a high resolution, double-focussing mass-spectrometer being necessary for many of the assays. For this reason, formally defined reference methods have been established to provide a link between the working laboratory and definitive assay technology. The IFCC define *reference methods* as: 'Methods which after exhaustive testing and comparison with a definitive method have been shown to have negligible inaccuracy'. The reference method is available to the working laboratory, the results it delivers for any given samples being accepted as a surrogate for the 'true values'. The results will inevitably be subject to some imprecision but this should be of a low order, the average of any set of repeated assays tending to the consensus 'true value', i.e. the value that would be obtained using the definitive method.

If the results delivered by a new assay method disagree with those of the reference method in any systematic way (e.g. always 10% higher), the new method is taken to be biased, i.e. inaccurate. Once this is established, steps can be taken to identify the source of the bias and perhaps correct it.

A fundamental prerequisite for the establishment of any definitive method is a detailed knowledge of the analyte, its structure, state and behaviour in the complicated test sample matrix. A large number of analytes certainly do not meet these requirements, proteins (and enzymes) and polypeptide hormones being typical. The problems of validating the 'accuracy' of assay methods for such analytes can be profound, particularly when the assay is directed at the biological *activity* of the analyte (a functional assay) rather than its structural properties (a structural assay). Many of the problems are well-known in the Bio-assay field and reference to the paper of Jerne and Wood can again be recommended.

10.2. A STUDY IN CONTINUITY

If no broad consensus is available (or possible) for the definitive assay of a particular analyte, the 'accuracy' of a new assay method can no longer be assessed simply in terms of a method comparison study. A number of *internal* methods of validation can be used—recovery studies, parallelism studies on test and calibration samples—but each have real limitations. In the final analysis, the correspondence of the assay results to the clinical condition of the patient may be the only realistic yardstick of 'accuracy', i.e. accuracy as a correspondence to the clinical 'truth'.

Nonetheless, the new method may be compared with alternative assay methods, the most obvious choice being the method currently employed in the analysts own laboratory. The strength's and weaknesses of this method should be well-known to the analyst from his own direct experience. If the new method is a candidate for replacing the existing method, the analyst is not so much concerned with accuracy as he is with continuity. The existing method is best referred to as a comparative method in the comparison study.

The comparative method has no valid claim to accuracy by consensus. A new method can be compared with the comparative method, but any systematic disagreement between their respective results on a common batch of test samples is of an entirely relative nature. Since neither method has a valid claim to the truth, they may agree completely and yet both be severely biased in an absolute sense, i.e. one method is as bad as the other.

The following story is attributed to Professor G. Harrison (quoted in Cohen et al., 1957) and has more to say about the method comparison study than any technical dissertation:

'A certain retired sea captain made his home in a secluded spot on the island of Zanzibar. As a sentimental reminder of his seafaring career he still had his ship's chronometer and religiously kept it wound and in good operating condition. Every day at exactly noon, as indicated on his chronometer, he observed the ritual of firing off a volley from a small cannon. On one rare occasion he received a visit from an old friend who inquired how the Captain verified the correctness of his chronometer. "Oh", he replied, "there is an horologist over there in the town of Zanzibar where I go whenever I lay in supplies. He has very reliable time and as I have fairly frequent occasion to go that way I almost always walk past his window and check my time against his". After his visit was over the visitor dropped into the horologist's shop and inquired how the horologist checked his time. "Oh", replied he, "there's an old sea-captain over on the other end of the island, who, I am told, is quite a fanatic about accurate time and who shoots off a gun every day exactly at noon, so I always check my time and correct it by his!" '

To summarize, we have two distinct interpretations of systematic disagreement between the results of two different assay methods for the same analyte:

1. If the 'reference' method employed has a national or international consensus for its accuracy (its correspondence to the truth if you like!), then any systematic difference between its results and those of a new assay method can be attributed to inaccuracy (or bias) in the new methodology, although definite steps should be taken to confirm that observation. A consensus is a 'state of the art' judgement and should not be held above question. Indeed, scientific progress ultimately depends upon the falsification of the prevailing consensus, given the qualification that you have something better to replace it with. The cynical

might argue that if enough experts can be found to agree upon a matter, it must be wrong!

2. If the 'reference' method has no consensus for its accuracy, i.e. it is a comparative method, then any systematic differences between its results and those of a new assay method are described as a relative bias. It cannot be ascribed to failings in either method since neither has any claim to represent the truth. The existence of a relative bias is important if it is intended that the new method, by virtue of its technical or economic advantages, is to replace the existing (comparative) method. Completely new reference intervals or normal values will have to be established for the new assay method prior to its routine use.

10.3. THE STATISTICAL PROBLEM

We have two sets of test results on a batch of test specimens, one set obtained using a reference method, or a comparative method, the other set using the new assay method. As a reasonable generalization, any systematic difference or bias between the two sets of values can be divided into two types, a constant bias and a proportional bias, as follows:

No bias		Constant bias (+10 mg/l)		Proportional bias (+10%)	
Ref.	New	Ref.	New	Ref.	New (%)
100	100	100	110	100	110
200	200	200	210	200	220
300	300	300	310	300	330
400	400	400	410	400	440

Note: the constant bias is expressed in the scale of measurement whilst the proportional bias is a percentage. If these values are plotted on a simple x–y graph (x = ref, y = new), the slope and y-intercept of a straight-line fitted to the data points reveals exactly the identity and magnitude of any bias present.

If *no bias* is present the estimated slope (b) will not be significantly different from 1 and the y-intercept (a) will not be significantly different from zero; *Fig. 55a.*

If a *constant bias* is present it will be reflected in the y-intercept, the value of which will be identical to the magnitude of the bias; *Fig. 55b*.

If a *proportional bias* is present, the slope *b* will differ significantly from 1·000, e.g. a proportional bias of −10% in the new method will produce a slope of 0·900 the difference from 1·000 being 0·1 or 10%; *Fig. 55c*.

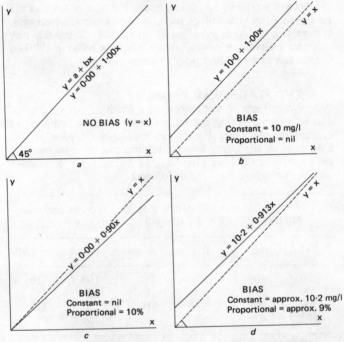

Fig. 55. Identification and quantification of systematic bias components in the method comparison study.

If both types of bias are present, the slope *b* and the *y*-intercept *a* will continue to differentiate and quantify the respective biases; *Fig. 55d*. So far we have chosen to overlook the imprecision or random (non-systematic) error of the assay methods. This evidences itself in the scatter of the points about the fitted line, the greater the imprecision of the methods, the greater the observed scatter.

The calculated slope (b) and y-intercept (a) are now sample statistics, subject to sampling uncertainty but, on average, consistent with the above interpretations.

The constant bias generally originates from inadequate blanking and as such is a relatively trivial technical problem. The proportional bias is of considerable importance since it is virtually undetectable outside of the method comparison study, unless it is so gross that the assay value clearly does not accord with the clinical reality. Tests of parallelism and recovery studies will not indicate its presence. It generally originates from inadequate calibration, i.e. the calibration material does not behave in an identical manner to the material in the test sample. If a pure hormone isolated from a cow's parathyroid glands is used to 'standardize' an assay for the analagous hormone in human serum, problems might be expected! If the hormone isolated from a human source is used, the extraction and isolation procedure may quite conceivably have altered its behaviour so that it no longer represents adequately the same hormone in its native state (in a test sample). Finally, there may be substances present in the test sample that are not found in the artificially prepared calibration standard(s), that behave in a similar manner to the test substance in the measurement system. The method is not *specific* for substance of interest. Wood (1948) had the following to say on this subject:

'If, for example, in a riboflavine assay the test preparation should happen to contain not only riboflavine, but also some other growth-stimulating factor, and if this other factor stimulated growth proportionally to the dosage at all dosage-levels, no statistical test and no method of calculating the result could possibly detect anything suspicious in the result obtained. The combined riboflavine and other factor would be estimated as riboflavine.'

The slope and intercept of the fitted straight line are commonly determined by the technique of least-squares, a simple linear regression model being implicitly assumed for the data. This technique for assessing the accuracy of assay values was described by Youden (1947) for application in the field of analytical chemistry, and he pointed out the necessity of observing the x-

variable without appreciable measurement error. Westgard and Hunt (1973) subsequently recommended the least-squares approach for the analysis of clinical chemical method-comparison studies. Clinical assay methods are generally a good deal more imprecise than pure analytical chemical assays and for the clinical method-comparison study, the x-variable (the reference method) cannot reasonably be assumed to be free from measurement errors. A casual inspection of published method-comparison studies is enough to reveal anything from 3 to 30% random errors in the comparative methods used.

It is a fundamental assumption of the simple linear regression model that the x-variable is free from random variation or measurement error.

Suppose that true values of the test specimens are represented by x_i. We obtain estimates of the x_i using a reference/comparative method and a new method:

$$\text{reference values: } \xi_i = x_i + \delta_i$$
$$\text{new values: } \quad \eta_i = y_i + \varepsilon_i \qquad (10.1)$$

ξ_i and η_i are the values we observe. The terms δ_i and ε_i are the random errors involved (measurement errors). The term y_i is the biased mean estimate of the new method, i.e., the true value x_i plus both a constant and a proportional bias:

$$y_i = \alpha + \beta x_i \qquad (10.2)$$

Recall the formula for estimating the least-squares slope b, from expression 8.7:

$$b = \frac{SS_{xy}}{SS_x} = \frac{\text{covariance } xy}{\text{variance } x} \qquad (8.7)$$

In the method comparison study, we do not observe x and y directly, but with additional measurement errors, as ξ and η.

$$b = \frac{\text{Covariance } \xi\eta}{\text{Variance } \xi} = \frac{\text{Covariance } xy}{\text{Variance } x + \text{Variance } \delta} \qquad (10.3)$$

If the measurement errors δ and ε are uncorrelated (a reasonable assumption for this case) the covariance of ξ and η decomposes to covariance xy. The lower term of expression 10.3 remains a compound of the variance of x (the true values) and the variance of δ (the measurement errors). The estimate of b from expression 10.3 will be lower than that from expression

8.7, the larger the measurement error in the reference method (variance δ), the lower the estimate will be.

The simple least squares model assumes that we have a reference method free from measurement errors, i.e. that the values it produces for test samples are x_i, not ξ_i. The model in this case is:

$$\eta_i = \alpha + \beta x_i + \varepsilon_i \tag{10.4}$$

Expression 8.7 is an unbiased estimator of β in this model.

The trouble is that we do *not* observe x_i, but ξ_i, for which we have the model:

$$\eta = \alpha + \beta \xi_i + (\varepsilon_i - \beta \delta_i) \tag{10.5}$$

Expression 8.7 is not an unbiased estimator of β for *this* model. The fact of the matter is that we are not dealing with a simple linear regression model at all, but a linear structural relation between x and y (expression 10.2) obscured by measurement errors in both variables (expression 10.5). Although this problem is being rediscovered by clinical chemists in the last few years, it is a well-known and much discussed problem in statistical circles with a history extending back at least to 1878 (Adcock).

10.4. THE ESTIMATION OF α AND β

If we can assume the random measurement errors of both assays to be at least approximately constant throughout the measurement range, the solution is relatively straightforward. We require one additional piece of information about the methods being compared, the *ratio* of their random error variances, λ, where:

$$\lambda = \frac{\text{Variance of error in new method}}{\text{Variance of error in reference method}} = \frac{S_\varepsilon^2}{S_\delta^2} \tag{10.6}$$

λ need not be exactly determined and estimates of the error variances from within-batch precision studies may be employed. A preferable source for the variance estimates is the method comparison study itself; if duplicate measurements (fully randomized) are made on every test specimen by each of the two assay methods involved, the error variances can be obtained (using the methods of *Table 8*) as follows in *Example 10.1*.

Example *10.1.*

Sample	Reference assay values				New assay values			
	ξ_1	ξ_2	$\bar{\bar{\xi}}$	$S_i{}^2$	η_1	η_2	$\bar{\eta}$	$S_i{}^2$
1	1606	1654	1628	1152	2009	1980	1994·5	420·5
2	180	215	197·5	612·5	240	258	249	162
3	1506	1479	1492·5	364·5	1699	1749	1724	1250
4	320	311	315·5	40·5	516	535	525·5	180·5
5	1130	1163	1146·5	544·5	1625	1595	1610	450
6	590	606	598	128	668	637	652·5	480·5
7	1318	1330	1324	72	1610	1588	1599	242
8	698	692	695	18	849	869	859	200
9	1148	1109	1125·5	760·5	1393	1355	1374	722
10	624	649	636·5	312·5	919	888	903·5	480·5
		means	915·9	400·5			means 1149·1	458·8

Note: $S_i{}^2 = (|\xi_1 - \xi_2|)/\sqrt{2})^2$, and similarly for η_1 and η_2.

Reference assay variance $= S_\delta{}^2 = 400·5$
New assay variance $\quad = S_\varepsilon{}^2 = 458·8$
$\lambda = 458·8/400·5 = 1·1456.$

The use of duplicate measurements in the comparison study is to be recommended providing as it does a ready check on the validity of any single assay value.

Calculations
Summations (using the means $\bar{\xi}_i$ and $\bar{\eta}_i$):

$$\Sigma\xi = 9159·0, \qquad\qquad \Sigma\eta = 11\ 491·0,$$
$$\Sigma\xi^2 = 10\ 596\ 436·5, \qquad \Sigma\eta^2 = 16\ 305\ 084·0,$$
$$\bar{\xi} = 915·9, \qquad\qquad\quad \eta = 1149·1,$$
$$\Sigma\xi\eta = 13\ 106\ 744·5, \qquad n = 10,$$

from which we obtain:

$$SS_\xi = \Sigma\xi^2 - (\Sigma\xi)^2/n = 2207\ 708·4,$$
$$SS_\eta = \Sigma\eta^2 - (\Sigma\eta)^2/n = 3100\ 775·9,$$
$$SS_{\xi\eta} = \Sigma\xi\eta - (\Sigma\xi)(\Sigma\eta)/n = 2\ 582\ 137·6.$$

Note: the correlation coefficient $r = SS_{\xi\eta}/\sqrt{SS_\xi \cdot SS_\eta}$
$= 0·9869.$

This quantity has no probabilistic interpretation in the context of a structural errors-in-variables model, as indicated in Chapter 8.

We are now in a position to calculate the slope and intercept of expression (10.5), as follows:

Calculate $\theta = SS_\eta - \lambda \cdot SS_\xi$
$$= 3100\ 775 \cdot 9 - (1 \cdot 1456 \times 2207\ 708 \cdot 4)$$
$$= 571\ 625 \cdot 157.$$

Calculate $\phi = 4 \cdot \lambda \cdot (SS_{\xi\eta})^2$
$$= 4 \times 1 \cdot 1456 \times (258\ 2137 \cdot 6)^2$$
$$= 3 \cdot 0553 \times 10^{13}.$$

$$\text{Slope } b = \frac{\theta + \sqrt{(\theta^2 + \phi)}}{2SS_{\xi\eta}} \tag{10.7}$$

$$= \frac{571\ 625 \cdot 157 + \sqrt{[(571\ 625 \cdot 157)^2 + 3 \cdot 0553 \times 10^{13}]}}{2 \times 2582\ 137 \cdot 6}$$

$$= 1 \cdot 1867.$$

$$y\text{-intercept } a = \bar{\eta} - b \cdot \bar{\xi} \tag{10.8}$$
$$= 1149 \cdot 1 - (1 \cdot 1867 \times 915 \cdot 9)$$
$$= 62 \cdot 18.$$

The line $\eta_i = 62 \cdot 18 + 1 \cdot 1867\xi_i$ can be fitted to a graph of the method comparison data quite simply. Insert a low and a high value of ξ into the equation and calculate the corresponding η values. The points are located on the graph and joined by a straight line. This should pass through the point defined by $\bar{\xi}, \bar{\eta}$ and should also cut the η axis at the value obtained for the intercept a above (*Fig. 56*).

10.5. CAUTIONS

The estimator of expression 10.7 assumes the random error variances of both assay methods to be reasonably constant throughout the measurement range considered. This is at least approximately true for many assays, but clearly untrue for many others. The estimator remains consistent in the presence of non-constant error variances (e.g. constant c.v. %) as long as the *ratio* of the error variances is not unduly disturbed, but it is less efficient, i.e. more test values are required to maintain the certainty with which the slope β is estimated.

If the error variances, or their ratio, are subject to marked variation throughout the concentration range, three courses of action present themselves.

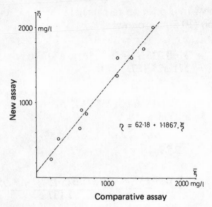

Fig. 56. Example 10.1.

1. You can employ a more sophisticated statistical analysis that takes account of the non-constant error variances by a procedure known as 'weighting'. Data points associated with large error-variances are given a low priority (a low weighting) in the analysis, since their 'information' content is relatively low, whilst data points associated with small error variances are given a high priority in the estimation of β.

The analysis requires estimates of the error variances associated with every data point. If a convenient relationship has been identified between the error variance and the concentration variable (e.g. from a dose precision profile; *see* Section 6.2), this can be employed directly in the weighting procedure. Failing this, it will be necessary to estimate the error variance associated with every assay value by replication of the test measurements, a minimum of ten replications (fully randomized) being essential if the weighted analysis is to exhibit any advantage at all over an unweighted analysis such as that of expression 10.7. The literature on the subject of weighted errors-in-variables models tends to be rather specialized (Bard, 1974) reflecting the complexity of the statistical problem.

2. A transformation of the test data may stabilize the error variances. For example, if the random error varies as a fixed percentage of the concentration value (i.e. a constant coefficient of variation) a logarithmic transformation of the assay values

will produce a constant error variance. The problem with this approach is that the constant and proportional bias components of the assay values are also transformed, severely distorting the error-structure of the data. As a general rule of thumb, transformations are best left in the hands of an experienced statistician; he will know where the quicksands are!

3. The third, and most practical, approach is a great deal simpler and not without certain advantages.

Rank the test values in ascending order of magnitude, based upon the mean reference assay values. Now divide the ranked values into three sub-groups, representing the low, mid-range and high concentration values. There is no need to have the same number of values in each group.

Proceed to analyze each sub-group exactly as if it were a complete comparison study in its own right. We are now assuming that the error-variances within each sub-group are less variable than they are across the entire sample group, to the extent that we may consider them approximately constant. This approach is not dissimilar to the biologists' 'broken-stick' model, i.e. approximating awkward relationships by a number of straight-line segments. It may prove quite adequate for your purposes and has the advantage of delivering the data for a ready-made dose-precision profile, i.e. a plot of the low, medium and high concentration range error variances against the corresponding sub-group means.

Given the possibility of having to fall back upon this 'broken-stick' model, it would pay to be selective about the specimens included in the original study group. Aim for a minimum of 150 test specimens, fifty low, fifty mid-range and fifty high analyte levels wherever this is possible.

The confidence interval for β described below is appropriate only when the assumption of a constant error variance ratio can be reasonably justified.

10.6. A 95% CONFIDENCE INTERVAL FOR THE SLOPE

The uncertainty in our slope estimate, b, arises from two main sources; from the random measurement errors in the test specimen responses; and from errors in the calibration of each assay method.

Maximum information on β is obtained by conducting the method comparison study over as many recalibrations of each assay method as possible. When all of the test specimens are processed in one or two batches to save time or effort, the price paid is maximal uncertainty in the estimate b. The data contains no 'information' on the effects of local calibration error. It makes sense. If you want a good indication of national opinion on a certain matter, you do not go out and ask one or two individuals the same question a hundred times, the exact equivalent of estimating calibration variation by assaying one hundred test specimens from one or two calibration curves.

The confidence intervals described below apply only to maximally recalibrated data, i.e. where every test result is accompanied by a recalibration of the assay.

$$95\% \text{ c.i. on } \beta = \sqrt{\lambda} \times \tan \left[\arctan (b/\sqrt{\lambda}) \pm Q\right], \quad (10.9)$$

$$\text{where } Q = 0 \cdot 5 \arcsin \left[2 \times t \sqrt{\left(\frac{\lambda \cdot (SS_\xi \cdot SS_\eta - (SS_{\xi\eta})^2)}{(n-2) \cdot (\theta^2 + \phi)} \right)} \right].$$

Don't allow yourself to be intimidated by expression 10.9. It is nothing more than simple (if tedious) arithmetic. The value for t is obtained from *Table F*, Appendix, reading down the left-hand column to $n - 2$ (for this example $n - 2 = 10 - 2 = 8$) and across to the column headed $0 \cdot 05$, i.e. $t = 2 \cdot 306$.

$$Q = 0 \cdot 5 \arcsin [2 \times 2 \cdot 306 \times$$
$$\sqrt{\left\{ \frac{1 \cdot 1456[(2207\ 708 \cdot 4 \times 3100\ 775 \cdot 9) - (2582\ 137 \cdot 6)^2]}{(10 - 2) \cdot ((571\ 625 \cdot 157)^2 + (3 \cdot 0553 \times 10^{13}))} \right\}} \right]$$

$$= 0 \cdot 5 \arcsin \left[2 \times 2 \cdot 306 \sqrt{\left(\frac{2 \cdot 0412 \times 10^{11}}{2 \cdot 4704 \times 10^{14}} \right)} \right]$$

$$= 3 \cdot 8091.$$

So we have:

$$95\% \text{ c.i. on } \beta =$$
$$\sqrt{1 \cdot 1456} \times \tan \left[\arctan (1 \cdot 1867/\sqrt{1 \cdot 1456}) \pm 3 \cdot 8901\right]$$
$$= 1 \cdot 0388 - 1 \cdot 3582.$$

Conclusions:

To summarize, we have:

$$\text{slope } b = 1 \cdot 1867 \ (95\% \text{ c.i.} = 1 \cdot 0388 - 1 \cdot 3582)$$

$$y\text{-intercept } a = 62 \cdot 18$$

The 95% c.i. on β excludes the value $1 \cdot 00$ so that we have some evidence to support the existence of a real proportional bias, the best single estimate of which is $(1 - 1 \cdot 1867) \times 100 = 18 \cdot 7\%$.

We have an estimate of $62 \cdot 18$ units for the constant bias. Is this evidence of real bias, or simply random sampling variation about a population bias of zero? The answer demands a little effort and is strictly confined to maximally recalibrated data.

First, let us estimate the between-batch error variances for each assay retrospectively, from the method comparison data itself:

new assay $s_\Delta^2 = (SS\eta - b \cdot SS\xi\eta)/(n - 2) = 4569 \cdot 15$

ref. assay $s_e^2 = s_\Delta^2/\lambda = 3988 \cdot 44$.

Using a result provided by Robertson (1974), we obtain the standard error of a as follows:

$$\text{s.e.} a = \sqrt{[(1/SS\xi) \cdot \{([(b^2 \cdot s_e^2) + s_\Delta^2][\bar{\xi}^2 + (SS\xi/n)]) + [(s_e^2 \cdot s_\Delta^2 \cdot \bar{\xi}^2)/(SS\xi/n)]\}.]}$$

Just respect the bracket priorities. For the test example we have a 95% c.i. on a of $a \pm [t_{n-2} \cdot \text{s.e.} a]$ which works out at $62 \cdot 18 \pm 162$. This range so clearly embraces the value zero that we have no good evidence to support the existence of a constant bias.

For the purpose of this elementary treatment of the method-comparison we have chosen to regard the random elements of the method-comparison model as being entirely due to measurement imprecision. There is a second source of 'scatter' attributable to *specimen dependent* non-specificity in the assay systems, e.g. interference and cross-reactions. The impact of these effects upon the estimate of λ (expression 10.6), and thus the slope and intercept estimates, has been treated as negligible. The effects are, however, fully accounted for in the confidence intervals described above.

The method comparison study has been set in the context of a method evaluation programme in *Table 16*. Guidelines to the conduct of such a programme have been published by the International Federation of Clinical Chemistry (Buttner et al., 1979).

Table 16. A framework for the evaluation of a new assay method

```
┌─────────────────────────┐
│ Transfer of base unit   │────── Parallelism studies
│ to secondary (in-house) │       with primary calibrator
│ calibrator              │
└─────────────────────────┘

┌─────────────────────────┐
│ *Parallelism* studies   │
│ with biological test    │
│ matrix                  │
└─────────────────────────┘

┌─────────────────────────┐
│ Response                │────── *Detection limit*
│ *precision components*  │────── Calibration curve:
│ profile                 │       goodness-of-fit
│                         │────── *Interference* studies
│                         │────── *Cross-reactivity* studies
└─────────────────────────┘

┌─────────────────────────┐
│ Dose                    │────── *Recovery studies*
│ *precision components*  │      ┌ Benchmark database for
│ profile                 │      │ assay *imprecision:*
│                         │      │ within-batch
│                         │      │ between-batch
└─────────────────────────┘      └ between-laboratory ──────┐
                                                             │
┌─────────────────────────┐                                 │
│ Method                  │                                 │
│ comparison studies      │────── Systematic bias           │
│                         │                                 │
└─────────────────────────┘                                 │

┌─────────────────────────┐                                 │
│ Interlaboratory         │────── *Clinical utility*         │
│ field studies           │      ┌ *Reference ranges*        │
│                         │      │ Normal                    │
│                         │      └ Pathologic                │
└─────────────────────────┘                                 │
        └────────────────────────────────────────────────────┘
```

REFERENCES

Adcock R. J. (1878) A problem in least squares. *The Analyst* 5, 53–55.

Bard Y. (1974) *Nonlinear Parameter Estimation*. New York, Academic.

Buttner J., Borth R., Boutwell J. H. et al. (1979) In: IFCC, Committee on Standards. Approved recommendation (1978) on quality control in clinical chemistry. Part 2, Assessment of analytical methods for routine use. *Clin. Chim. Acta* 98, 145F–162F.

Cohen E. R., Crowe K. M. and Dumond J. W. M. (1957) *Fundamental Constants in Physics*. New York, Interscience p. iv.

Jerne N. K. and Wood E. C. (1949) The validity and meaning of the results of biological assays. *Biometrics* 5, 273–299.

Robertson C. A. (1974) Large sample theory for the linear structural relation. *Biometrika* 61, pp. 353–359.

Westgard J. O. and Hunt M. R. (1973) Use and interpretation of common statistical tests in method comparison studies. *Clin. Chem.* 19, 49–57.

Wood E. C. (1948) The theory of certain analytical procedures with particular reference to microbiological assays. *The Analyst* 71, 1–14.

Youden W. J. (1947) Technique for testing the accuracy of analytical data. *An. Chem.* 19, 946–950.

An advanced treatment of the errors-in-variables models can be found in the following texts:

Kendall M. G. and Stuart A. (1973) *The Advanced Theory of Statistics* vol. 2. London & High Wycombe, Griffin.

Sprent P. (1969) *Models in Regression and Related Topics*. London, Methuen.

11 Final Thoughts

1. Formulate your question exactly. Just what is it you want to know?

2. Find out what sort of data you need, how much of it you need and how to collect it. A statistician can help you here and may additionally be of real help in formulating your question exactly. He may suggest a suitable experimental design to simplify the analysis and increase the probability of obtaining an unambiguous answer to your question.

3. Collect and analyse the data. The technique of analysis will be determined at stage two, before the data is collected.

4. Ask yourself if the results actually make sense. If they do not, either the statistical analysis is at fault (faulty arithmetic, unjustified assumptions, unrepresentative sample) or—you have made a discovery . . . .

5. Be sure you publish only your discoveries . . . .

Appendix: Tables A - G

Table A. Random digits

938	460	624	277	995	274	984	186	657	492	505	903	648	876	414
543	156	843	303	858	563	534	775	648	319	863	829	480	646	495
724	833	958	666	204	785	311	157	789	925	207	517	242	630	851
633	497	371	480	243	716	279	783	790	610	441	380	904	689	277
139	347	946	462	410	172	696	327	412	570	813	806	177	601	239
572	543	326	519	154	789	748	129	488	118	290	651	633	246	731
864	783	164	825	473	850	164	918	500	880	218	712	427	337	275
115	253	237	670	795	831	639	702	224	936	652	976	971	169	646
716	143	955	930	644	163	885	572	193	253	336	554	410	982	322
932	243	984	379	968	445	713	607	164	424	818	971	221	636	322
379	790	746	446	480	843	120	108	353	857	487	263	451	549	518
421	137	398	759	229	317	336	425	599	265	663	842	822	806	526
352	950	409	420	171	532	833	872	735	645	256	876	877	921	665
400	729	104	134	670	645	625	706	963	876	819	964	737	895	974
755	339	474	800	278	849	557	356	372	565	911	566	961	811	456
446	238	706	588	630	858	805	844	520	854	974	233	576	176	711
559	625	110	953	960	321	867	756	825	210	754	630	862	173	565
343	511	113	881	178	930	395	663	156	673	138	750	226	860	939
255	187	199	233	488	303	556	128	292	946	177	615	656	947	821
989	162	287	423	302	603	855	463	765	111	494	361	361	700	225
157	359	442	615	596	108	146	311	232	139	457	491	517	945	279
479	134	325	622	625	407	315	193	482	127	378	451	167	182	248
333	521	863	789	100	336	445	275	354	456	487	981	958	357	853
913	301	429	728	516	816	774	260	630	540	514	906	101	810	214
851	176	377	863	537	481	663	924	192	257	302	766	639	269	344
932	680	254	850	457	497	297	691	954	562	647	337	836	841	992
299	797	907	426	899	165	183	934	684	202	892	550	329	694	764
755	420	476	128	351	771	386	466	839	859	300	167	892	885	522
335	186	575	841	822	894	737	793	514	733	337	594	214	807	196
780	249	395	745	204	316	304	317	764	570	359	231	905	924	473

Table B. Areas under the Normal distribution curve.

z	0	1	2	3	4	5	6	7	8	9
0·0	0·0000	0·0040	0·0080	0·0120	0·0160	0·0199	0·0239	0·0279	0·0319	0·0359
0·1	0·0398	0·0438	0·0478	0·0517	0·0557	0·0596	0·0636	0·0675	0·0714	0·0753
0·2	0·0793	0·0832	0·0871	0·0910	0·0948	0·0987	0·1026	0·1064	0·1103	0·1141
0·3	0·1179	0·1217	0·1255	0·1293	0·1331	0·1368	0·1406	0·1443	0·1480	0·1517
0·4	0·1554	0·1591	0·1628	0·1664	0·1700	0·1736	0·1772	0·1808	0·1844	0·1879
0·5	0·1915	0·1950	0·1985	0·2019	0·2054	0·2088	0·2123	0·2157	0·2190	0·2224
0·6	0·2257	0·2291	0·2324	0·2357	0·2389	0·2422	0·2454	0·2486	0·2517	0·2549
0·7	0·2580	0·2611	0·2642	0·2673	0·2704	0·2734	0·2764	0·2794	0·2823	0·2852
0·8	0·2881	0·2910	0·2939	0·2967	0·2995	0·3023	0·3051	0·3078	0·3106	0·3133
0·9	0·3159	0·3186	0·3212	0·3238	0·3264	0·3289	0·3315	0·3340	0·3365	0·3389
1·0	0·3413	0·3438	0·3461	0·3485	0·3508	0·3531	0·3554	0·3577	0·3599	0·3621
1·1	0·3643	0·3665	0·3686	0·3708	0·3729	0·3749	0·3770	0·3790	0·3810	0·3830
1·2	0·3849	0·3869	0·3888	0·3907	0·3925	0·3944	0·3962	0·3980	0·3997	0·4015
1·3	0·4032	0·4049	0·4066	0·4082	0·4099	0·4115	0·4131	0·4147	0·4162	0·4177
1·4	0·4192	0·4207	0·4222	0·4236	0·4251	0·4265	0·4279	0·4292	0·4306	0·4319
1·5	0·4332	0·4345	0·4357	0·4370	0·4382	0·4394	0·4406	0·4418	0·4429	0·4441
1·6	0·4452	0·4463	0·4474	0·4484	0·4495	0·4505	0·4515	0·4525	0·4535	0·4545
1·7	0·4554	0·4564	0·4573	0·4582	0·4591	0·4599	0·4608	0·4616	0·4625	0·4633
1·8	0·4641	0·4649	0·4656	0·4664	0·4671	0·4678	0·4686	0·4693	0·4699	0·4706
1·9	0·4713	0·4719	0·4726	0·4732	0·4738	0·4744	0·4750	0·4756	0·4761	0·4767
2·0	0·4772	0·4778	0·4783	0·4788	0·4793	0·4798	0·4803	0·4808	0·4812	0·4817
2·1	0·4821	0·4826	0·4830	0·4834	0·4838	0·4842	0·4846	0·4850	0·4854	0·4857
2·2	0·4861	0·4864	0·4868	0·4871	0·4875	0·4878	0·4881	0·4884	0·4887	0·4890
2·3	0·4893	0·4896	0·4898	0·4901	0·4904	0·4906	0·4909	0·4911	0·4913	0·4916
2·4	0·4918	0·4920	0·4922	0·4925	0·4927	0·4929	0·4931	0·4932	0·4934	0·4936
2·5	0·4938	0·4940	0·4941	0·4943	0·4945	0·4946	0·4948	0·4949	0·4951	0·4952
2·6	0·4953	0·4955	0·4956	0·4957	0·4959	0·4960	0·4961	0·4962	0·4963	0·4964
2·7	0·4965	0·4966	0·4967	0·4968	0·4969	0·4970	0·4971	0·4972	0·4973	0·4974
2·8	0·4974	0·4975	0·4976	0·4977	0·4977	0·4978	0·4979	0·4979	0·4980	0·4981
2·9	0·4981	0·4982	0·4982	0·4983	0·4984	0·4984	0·4985	0·4985	0·4986	0·4986
3·0	0·4987	0·4987	0·4987	0·4988	0·4988	0·4989	0·4989	0·4989	0·4990	0·4990
3·1	0·4990	0·4991	0·4991	0·4991	0·4992	0·4992	0·4992	0·4992	0·4993	0·4993
3·2	0·4993	0·4993	0·4994	0·4994	0·4994	0·4994	0·4994	0·4995	0·4995	0·4995
3·3	0·4995	0·4995	0·4995	0·4996	0·4996	0·4996	0·4996	0·4996	0·4996	0·4997
3·4	0·4997	0·4997	0·4997	0·4997	0·4997	0·4997	0·4997	0·4997	0·4997	0·4998
3·5	0·4998	0·4998	0·4998	0·4998	0·4998	0·4998	0·4998	0·4998	0·4998	0·4998

Source: Generated by author using Hewlett-Packard HP-41c applications module HP 00041-15002.

Table C. Critical values of the Kolmogorov–Smirnov test statistic *d*-max (unknown mean and variance)

n	5%	1%
4	0·381	0·417
5	0·337	0·405
6	0·319	0·364
7	0·300	0·348
8	0·285	0·331
9	0·271	0·311
10	0·258	0·294
11	0·249	0·284
12	0·242	0·275
13	0·234	0·268
14	0·227	0·261
15	0·220	0·257
16	0·213	0·250
17	0·206	0·245
18	0·200	0·239
19	0·195	0·235
20	0·190	0·231
25	0·180	0·203
30	0·161	0·187
Over 30	$\dfrac{0 \cdot 886}{\sqrt{N}}$	$\dfrac{1 \cdot 031}{\sqrt{N}}$

Source: Condensed from H. W. Lilliefors (1967). On the Kolmogorov–Smirnov test for Normality with mean and variance unknown. *J. Am. Statis. Ass.* **62,** 399–402. Reproduced with the permission of the American Statistical Association.

Table D. Critical values of the Kolmogorov–Smirnov test statistic d-max, (mean and variance known)

n	5%	1%	n	5%	1%	n	5%	1%	n	5%	1%	n	5%	1%
1	0·9750	0·9950	21	0·2872	0·3443	41	0·2076	0·2490	61	0·1709	0·2051	81	0·1487	0·1784
2	0·8419	0·9293	22	0·2809	0·3367	42	0·2052	0·2461	62	0·1696	0·2034	82	0·1478	0·1773
3	0·7076	0·8290	23	0·2749	0·3295	43	0·2028	0·2433	63	0·1682	0·2018	83	0·1469	0·1763
4	0·6239	0·7342	24	0·2693	0·3229	44	0·2006	0·2406	64	0·1669	0·2003	84	0·1460	0·1752
5	0·5633	0·6685	25	0·2640	0·3166	45	0·1984	0·2380	65	0·1657	0·1988	85	0·1452	0·1742
6	0·5193	0·6166	26	0·2591	0·3106	46	0·1963	0·2354	66	0·1644	0·1973	86	0·1444	0·1732
7	0·4834	0·5758	27	0·2544	0·3050	47	0·1942	0·2330	67	0·1632	0·1958	87	0·1435	0·1722
8	0·4543	0·5418	28	0·2499	0·2997	48	0·1922	0·2306	68	0·1620	0·1944	88	0·1427	0·1713
9	0·4300	0·5133	29	0·2457	0·2947	49	0·1903	0·2283	69	0·1609	0·1930	89	0·1419	0·1703
10	0·4092	0·4889	30	0·2417	0·2899	50	0·1884	0·2260	70	0·1597	0·1917	90	0·1412	0·1694
11	0·3912	0·4677	31	0·2379	0·2853	51	0·1866	0·2239	71	0·1586	0·1903	91	0·1404	0·1685
12	0·3754	0·4490	32	0·2342	0·2809	52	0·1848	0·2217	72	0·1576	0·1890	92	0·1396	0·1676
13	0·3614	0·4325	33	0·2308	0·2768	53	0·1831	0·2197	73	0·1565	0·1878	93	0·1389	0·1667
14	0·3489	0·4176	34	0·2274	0·2728	54	0·1814	0·2177	74	0·1554	0·1865	94	0·1382	0·1658
15	0·3376	0·4042	35	0·2242	0·2690	55	0·1798	0·2157	75	0·1544	0·1853	95	0·1375	0·1649
16	0·3273	0·3920	36	0·2212	0·2653	56	0·1782	0·2138	76	0·1534	0·1841	96	0·1368	0·1641
17	0·3180	0·3809	37	0·2183	0·2618	57	0·1767	0·2120	77	0·1524	0·1829	97	0·1361	0·1632
18	0·3094	0·3706	38	0·2154	0·2584	58	0·1752	0·2102	78	0·1515	0·1817	98	0·1354	0·1624
19	0·3014	0·3612	39	0·2127	0·2552	59	0·1737	0·2084	79	0·1505	0·1806	99	0·1347	0·1616
20	0·2941	0·3524	40	0·2101	0·2521	60	0·1723	0·2067	80	0·1496	0·1795	100	0·1340	0·1608

Source: Reproduced by permission of George Allen & Unwin from *Statistics Tables* (1978) by H. R. Neave.

Table E. Critical values of the linear
correlation coefficient

n	0·05	0·01
5	0·878	0·959
6	0·811	0·917
7	0·754	0·875
8	0·707	0·834
9	0·666	0·798
10	0·632	0·765
11	0·602	0·735
12	0·576	0·708
13	0·553	0·684
14	0·532	0·661
15	0·514	0·641
16	0·497	0·623
17	0·482	0·606
18	0·468	0·590
19	0·456	0·575
20	0·444	0·561
25	0·396	0·505
30	0·361	0·463
40	0·312	0·403
50	0·279	0·361
60	0·254	0·330
70	0·235	0·306
80	0·220	0·286
90	0·207	0·270
100	0·197	0·256
200	0·139	0·182

Table F. Student's *t* distribution

	Probability of a deviation greater than *t* (two-sided)			
$n-1$	0·10	0·05	0·02	0·01
1	6·314	12·706	31·821	63·657
2	2·920	4·303	6·965	9·925
3	2·353	3·182	4·541	5·841
4	2·132	2·776	3·747	4·604
5	2·015	2·571	3·365	4·032
6	1·943	2·447	3·143	3·707
7	1·895	2·365	2·998	3·499
8	1·860	2·306	2·896	3·355
9	1·833	2·262	2·821	3·250
10	1·812	2·228	2·764	3·169
11	1·796	2·201	2·718	3·106
12	1·782	2·179	2·681	3·055
13	1·771	2·160	2·650	3·012
14	1·761	2·145	2·624	2·977
15	1·753	2·131	2·602	2·947
16	1·746	2·120	2·583	2·921
17	1·740	2·110	2·567	2·898
18	1·734	2·101	2·552	2·878
19	1·729	2·093	2·539	2·861
20	1·725	2·086	2·528	2·845
21	1·721	2·080	2·518	2·831
22	1·717	2·074	2·508	2·819
23	1·714	2·069	2·500	2·807
24	1·711	2·064	2·492	2·797
25	1·708	2·060	2·485	2·787
26	1·706	2·056	2·479	2·770
27	1·703	2·052	2·473	2·771
28	1·701	2·048	2·467	2·763
29	1·699	2·045	2·462	2·756
30	1·697	2·042	2·457	2·750
40	1·684	2·021	2·423	2·704
60	1·671	2·000	2·390	2·660
120	1·658	1·980	2·358	2·617
∞	1·645	1·960	2·326	2·576

Table G. Normal scores and the sums of their squares
Part A.

Normal scores, $n = 1$–30.

r	n 1	2	3	4	5	6	7	8	9	10
1	0·0000	0·5642	0·8463	1·0294	1·1630	1·2672	1·3522	1·4236	1·4850	1·5388
2		0·0000	0·2970	0·4950	0·6418	0·7574	0·8522	0·9323	1·0014
3			0·0000	0·2015	0·3527	0·4728	0·5720	0·6561
4				0·0000	0·1525	0·2745	0·3758
5					0·0000	0·1227

r	n 11	12	13	14	15	16	17	18	19	20
1	1·5864	1·6292	1·6680	1·7034	1·7359	1·7660	1·7939	1·8200	1·8445	1·8675
2	1·0619	1·1157	1·1641	1·2079	1·2479	1·2847	1·3188	1·3504	1·3799	1·4076
3	0·7288	0·7928	0·8498	0·9011	0·9477	0·9903	1·0295	1·0657	1·0995	1·1309
4	0·4620	0·5368	0·6029	0·6618	0·7149	0·7632	0·8074	0·8481	0·8859	0·9210
5	0·2249	0·3122	0·3883	0·4556	0·5157	0·5700	0·6195	0·6648	0·7066	0·7454
6	0·0000	0·1026	0·1905	0·2673	0·3353	0·3962	0·4513	0·5016	0·5477	0·5903
7		0·0000	0·0882	0·1653	0·2338	0·2952	0·3508	0·4016	0·4483
8			0·0000	0·0773	0·1460	0·2077	0·2637	0·3149
9				0·0000	0·0688	0·1307	0·1870
10					0·0000	0·0620

r	n 21	22	23	24	25	26	27	28	29	30
1	1·8892	1·9097	1·9292	1·9477	1·9653	1·9822	1·9983	2·0137	2·0285	2·0428
2	1·4336	1·4582	1·4814	1·5034	1·5243	1·5442	1·5633	1·5815	1·5989	1·6156
3	1·1605	1·1882	1·2144	1·2392	1·2628	1·2851	1·3064	1·3267	1·3462	1·3648
4	0·9538	0·9846	1·0136	1·0409	1·0668	1·0914	1·1147	1·1370	1·1582	1·1786
5	0·7815	0·8153	0·8470	0·8768	0·9050	0·9317	0·9570	0·9812	1·0041	1·0261
6	0·6298	0·6667	0·7012	0·7335	0·7641	0·7929	0·8202	0·8462	0·8708	0·8944
7	0·4915	0·5316	0·5690	0·6040	0·6369	0·6679	0·6973	0·7251	0·7515	0·7767
8	0·3620	0·4056	0·4461	0·4839	0·5193	0·5527	0·5841	0·6138	0·6420	0·6689
9	0·2384	0·2858	0·3297	0·3705	0·4086	0·4444	0·4780	0·5098	0·5398	0·5683
10	0·1184	0·1700	0·2175	0·2616	0·3027	0·3410	0·3771	0·4110	0·4430	0·4733
11	0·0000	0·0564	0·1081	0·1558	0·2001	0·2413	0·2798	0·3160	0·3501	0·3824
12		0·0000	0·0518	0·0995	0·1439	0·1852	0·2239	0·2602	0·2945
13			0·0000	0·0478	0·0922	0·1336	0·1724	0·2088
14				0·0000	0·0444	0·0859	0·1247
15					0·0000	0·0415

Sums of squares of normal scores, $\sum_{i=1}^{n} S_i^2$ for $n = 1$–30.

Part B.

n	ΣS_i^2	n	ΣS_i^2	n	ΣS_i^2	n	ΣS_i^2	n	ΣS_i^2	n	ΣS_i^2
1	0·00000	6	4·11657	11	8·87931	16	13·74974	21	18·66306	26	23·59894
2	0·63662	7	5·05281	12	9·84812	17	14·72990	22	19·64880	27	24·58795
3	1·43239	8	5·99949	13	10·82002	18	15·71147	23	20·63534	28	25·57745
4	2·29566	9	6·95392	14	11·79451	19	16·69428	24	21·62258	29	26·56741
5	3·19506	10	7·91427	15	12·77119	20	17·67818	25	22·61046	30	27·55779

Table G. (continued)

Part A.

Normal scores, n = 31—50.

r	n 31	32	33	34	35	36	37	38	39	40
1	2·0565	2·0697	2·0824	2·0947	2·1066	2·1181	2·1293	2·1401	2·1506	2·1608
2	1·6317	1·6471	1·6620	1·6764	1·6902	1·7036	1·7166	1·7291	1·7413	1·7531
3	1·3827	1·3998	1·4164	1·4323	1·4476	1·4624	1·4768	1·4906	1·5040	1·5170
4	1·1980	1·2167	1·2347	1·2520	1·2686	1·2847	1·3002	1·3151	1·3296	1·3437
5	1·0471	1·0672	1·0865	1·1051	1·1230	1·1402	1·1568	1·1728	1·1883	1·2033
6	0·9169	0·9384	0·9590	0·9789	0·9979	1·0162	1·0339	1·0509	1·0674	1·0833
7	0·8007	0·8236	0·8455	0·8666	0·8868	0·9063	0·9250	0·9430	0·9604	0·9772
8	0·6944	0·7187	0·7420	0·7643	0·7857	0·8063	0·8261	0·8451	0·8634	0·8811
9	0·5955	0·6213	0·6460	0·6695	0·6921	0·7138	0·7346	0·7547	0·7740	0·7926
10	0·5021	0·5294	0·5555	0·5804	0·6043	0·6271	0·6490	0·6701	0·6904	0·7099
11	0·4129	0·4418	0·4694	0·4957	0·5208	0·5449	0·5679	0·5900	0·6113	0·6318
12	0·3269	0·3575	0·3867	0·4144	0·4409	0·4662	0·4904	0·5136	0·5359	0·5574
13	0·2432	0·2757	0·3065	0·3358	0·3637	0·3903	0·4158	0·4401	0·4635	0·4859
14	0·1613	0·1957	0·2283	0·2592	0·2886	0·3166	0·3434	0·3689	0·3934	0·4169
15	0·0804	0·1169	0·1515	0·1841	0·2151	0·2446	0·2727	0·2995	0·3252	0·3498
16	0·0000	0·0389	0·0755	0·1101	0·1428	0·1739	0·2034	0·2316	0·2585	0·2842
17			0·0000	0·0366	0·0712	0·1040	0·1351	0·1647	0·1929	0·2199
18					0·0000	0·0346	0·0674	0·0985	0·1282	0·1564
19							0·0000	0·0328	0·0640	0·0936
20									0·0000	0·0312

r	n 41	42	43	44	45	46	47	48	49	50
1	2·1707	2·1803	2·1897	2·1988	2·2077	2·2164	2·2249	2·2331	2·2412	2·2491
2	1·7646	1·7757	1·7865	1·7971	1·8073	1·8173	1·8271	1·8366	1·8458	1·8549
3	1·5296	1·5419	1·5538	1·5653	1·5766	1·5875	1·5982	1·6086	1·6187	1·6286
4	1·3573	1·3705	1·3833	1·3957	1·4078	1·4196	1·4311	1·4422	1·4531	1·4637
5	1·2178	1·2319	1·2456	1·2588	1·2717	1·2842	1·2964	1·3083	1·3198	1·3311
6	1·0987	1·1136	1·1281	1·1421	1·1558	1·1690	1·1819	1·1944	1·2066	1·2185
7	0·9935	1·0092	1·0245	1·0392	1·0536	1·0675	1·0810	1·0942	1·1070	1·1195
8	0·8982	0·9148	0·9308	0·9463	0·9614	0·9760	0·9902	1·0040	1·0174	1·0304
9	0·8106	0·8279	0·8447	0·8610	0·8767	0·8920	0·9068	0·9213	0·9353	0·9489
10	0·7287	0·7469	0·7645	0·7815	0·7979	0·8139	0·8294	0·8444	0·8590	0·8732
11	0·6515	0·6705	0·6889	0·7067	0·7238	0·7405	0·7566	0·7723	0·7875	0·8023
12	0·5780	0·5979	0·6171	0·6356	0·6535	0·6709	0·6877	0·7040	0·7198	0·7351
13	0·5075	0·5283	0·5483	0·5676	0·5863	0·6044	0·6219	0·6388	0·6552	0·6712
14	0·4394	0·4611	0·4820	0·5022	0·5217	0·5405	0·5586	0·5763	0·5933	0·6099
15	0·3734	0·3960	0·4178	0·4389	0·4591	0·4787	0·4976	0·5159	0·5336	0·5508
16	0·3089	0·3326	0·3553	0·3772	0·3983	0·4187	0·4383	0·4573	0·4757	0·4935
17	0·2457	0·2704	0·2942	0·3170	0·3390	0·3602	0·3806	0·4003	0·4194	0·4379
18	0·1835	0·2093	0·2341	0·2579	0·2808	0·3029	0·3241	0·3446	0·3644	0·3836
19	0·1219	0·1490	0·1749	0·1997	0·2236	0·2465	0·2686	0·2899	0·3105	0·3304
20	0·0608	0·0892	0·1163	0·1422	0·1671	0·1910	0·2140	0·2361	0·2575	0·2781
21	0·0000	0·0297	0·0580	0·0851	0·1111	0·1360	0·1599	0·1830	0·2051	0·2265
22			0·0000	0·0283	0·0555	0·0814	0·1064	0·1303	0·1534	0·1756
23					0·0000	0·0271	0·0531	0·0781	0·1020	0·1251
24							0·0000	0·0260	0·0509	0·0749
25									0·0000	0·0250

Sums of squares of normal scores, n = 31—50.

Part B.

n	ΣS_t^2	n	ΣS_t^2	n	ΣS_t^2	n	ΣS_t^2
31	28·54856	36	33·50736	41	38·47268	46	43·44284
32	29·53969	37	34·49997	42	39·46636	47	44·43735
33	30·53116	38	35·49282	43	40·46023	48	45·43200
34	31·52294	39	36·48589	44	41·45427	49	46·42678
35	32·51501	40	37·47918	45	42·44848	50	47·42170

Source: Reproduced by permission of George Allen & Unwin from *Statistics Tables* (1978) by H. R. Neave.

Index